**Maggie Jones** is a freelance journalist who has written for the *Guardian*, the *Observer*, the *Independent*, *Best* and *Parents* and is the author of twelve books, mainly on health and childcare issues. She is also a trained counsellor. She lives in London with her husband and three children.

YOUR CHILD SERIES

A series of books containing easy-to-follow, practical advice for the parents of children with a variety of illnesses or conditions.

Each book provides a clear overview of the situation, explaining essential information about the illness or condition and outlining the practical steps parents can take to help understand, support and care for their child, the rest of the family as well as themselves. Guiding parents through the conventional, the complementary and the alternative approaches available, these books cater for children of all ages, ranging from babies to teenagers, and enable the whole family to move forward in a positive way.

Other books in the series:

*Your Child: Asthma* by Erika Harvey
*Your Child: Bullying* by Jenny Alexander
*Your Child: Diabetes* by Catherine Steven

# YOUR CHILD

# Eczema

## Practical and Easy-to-Follow Advice

Maggie Jones

ELEMENT

Shaftesbury, Dorset • Boston, Massachusetts
Melbourne, Victoria

© Element Books Limited 1998
Text © Maggie Jones 1998

First published in Great Britain in 1998 by
Element Books Limited
Shaftesbury, Dorset SP7 8BP

Published in the USA in 1998 by
Element Books, Inc.
160 North Washington Street
Boston, MA 02114

Published in Australia in 1998 by
Element Books and distributed
by Penguin Books Australia Ltd
487 Maroondah Highway, Ringwood,
Victoria 3134

Design by Roger Lightfoot
Typeset by Bournemouth Colour Press, Parkstone
Printed and bound in Great Britain by Creative Print & Design, Wales

British Library Cataloguing in Publication
data available

Library of Congress Cataloging in Publication
data available

ISBN 1 86204 209 8

# Contents

# Introduction

Eczema is a common condition which affects as many as one in eight babies and young children. It is a red, scaly, itchy rash which causes flaking of the skin which may weep and form a crust. Areas of hard, thick skin can form from continual scratching, and the skin can become broken and prone to infection. At its worst eczema can be disfiguring and can cause great distress both to the child, who suffers from constant itching, and to the parents, who have to deal with this.

The word 'eczema' comes from a Greek word which means 'to boil over' which is a good description of how a child with severe eczema feels. The hot, itchy rash can seem unbearable, and it is very hard for young children to restrain themselves from scratching and making the skin worse.

Like many allergic conditions, eczema seems to be on the increase. This may be because of the increasing number of artificial chemicals in the environment, which may affect the skin. Recent surveys have also shown that many modern children have a poor diet, lacking in vitamins and with many artificial additives which may provoke allergic reactions. Schoolchildren frequently skip meals and make do with chocolate or fatty snacks, and they may go short of vitamin B in particular, which is needed for healthy skin. Also, breast-feeding protects against eczema and in our modern society only a very small number of babies receive no cow's milk formula or other artificial milks in the first six months of life.

The tendency to eczema is usually inherited, so if either parent suffered from eczema as a child, your child's chances of developing it are greater. If you suffered from eczema as a child, you will probably sympathize, but you may have forgotten the problems it caused you and think that your child will simply grow out of it as you did. Of course children do grow out of it, but they can still suffer a great deal along the way, and there is a lot you can do to help stop the condition worsening or even prevent it developing at all; at the very least, you can alleviate your child's distress.

People who have never suffered from eczema tend to think of it as a trivial complaint, but this is far from being the case. Eczema in a young baby can cause irritable, fractious behaviour and sleeplessness, and add greatly to the stresses everyone feels on becoming a parent. Further, eczema can spoil your baby's appearance and lead to embarrassment. Everyone likes to look at a new baby, but if every time strangers look they ask, 'What is that rash?' or 'What's wrong with him?' it can be very distressing and make you feel that you have failed in not producing a 'perfect' baby.

A baby who wakes frequently at night hot, itching and crying inconsolably will soon drive any parent into a state of exhaustion and distraction. As your child grows, poor sleep may become a fact of life and may also become a habit which can be very difficult to break. The combination of exhausted parents and tired, fractious toddler can make the joys of parenthood very hard to appreciate.

As your child gets older, eczema can mark him or her out from others at school and continue to be a source of stress for the whole family, causing irritability and bad temper and interfering with relationships. Brothers or sisters may resent the additional attention that their sibling receives and behave badly to gain attention and try to get you to prove that you love them just as much. Primary school children may feel different from their peers and find it harder to make friends, and teenagers with eczema may suffer dreadfully from shyness and loss of confidence, especially if the rash affects the face.

Constant itching is as bad as being in pain and sufferers may be irritable and have problems concentrating. This, together with poor sleep, can make it difficult for your child to achieve well in school, as can loss of confidence.

A recent survey among 4,000 members of the National Eczema Society in the UK revealed that 60 per cent of parents said that their children's sleep was affected by eczema, 27 per cent felt that sporting activities had been restricted, 25 per cent said that holidays were affected, school attendance was down in 15 per cent of children, and 14 per cent reported that their children's eczema affected their ability to play and meet other children.

Changes in diet can be irksome enough to an adult, but with children it can be distressing and often difficult to enforce. Children cannot always understand that certain foods make their eczema worse and are tempted to eat forbidden foods, especially at parties or when out of sight of their parents. The child who is forbidden chocolates, sweets and ice creams will often feel unloved and left out, and be envious of other children who are allowed to have such treats. Older children are sometimes teased or taunted by their peers for refusing foods to which they react badly.

While the conventional medicines given to treat eczema, such as steroids and antihistamines, may relieve the symptoms, they can have serious adverse effects on children. Steroids are linked to hyperactivity and difficulty in concentrating, and they tend to become less effective the more they are used, as the body develops a resistance to them. Higher doses tend to be needed to control the eczema, therefore, and can eventually reach harmful levels – excessively high levels of steroids can have damaging effects, leading to acne, hormone imbalances and stunted growth. Antihistamines can make children drowsy, so the 'cure' can cause as many problems as it causes. And other medical treatments, such a bandaging the child with bandages containing special creams, can seem almost barbaric.

Alternative medicines and health treatments have begun to be recognized as being of great benefit to sufferers of eczema.

Homoeopathy, acupuncture, herbal medicines and other natural remedies have become increasingly widely available and provide an alternative to conventional medicine. Indeed, Chinese herbal medicine has been so successful that Great Ormond Street Hospital for Children in the UK now refers children with severe eczema which does not respond to conventional treatment to registered herbal practitioners. Some of their treatments have been particularly successful with children, and have done much to relieve the symptoms.

Parents of children with eczema usually have to pay far more attention to their children's diet, lifestyle and environment than other parents. Because house-dust mites are a common cause of eczema, many parents have to vacuum, dust and generally clean their house, and especially their child's bedroom, far more often than others, as well as washing their clothes and bedclothes frequently. Since bad eczema leaves the skin raw and open to infections, it is obviously very important that your home, especially your kitchen and bathroom, are clean so that harmful household germs are kept to a minimum. You may also need to make sure that your child's skin is covered during outdoor play.

Your child's skin has to be kept clean, so baths are more frequent, and special cleaning agents have to be used instead of soap. The skin will need to be rubbed with aqueous or other creams at least once or twice a day, especially in the affected areas, and the bedtime ritual can take ages. Special foods have to be bought and prepared and vigilance is required to make sure that your child is not eating forbidden foods when your back is turned.

But while it is obviously important to take care of your child's diet and to keep the house clean, some parents of children with eczema can become so obsessed with cleanliness and diet that their children's lives become a misery; they cannot go to parties because they cannot eat the food, they cannot stay overnight with other people because they will not be able to cope, and so on. It is important that you do not let this happen to you, and let your child's life be as normal as possible. You can provide substitute foods as a matter of course so that your child does not feel left out, even when guests come – if there is a problem with cow's milk, for example, you can buy goat or sheep's milk yoghurt which you can sweeten with fruit purée, and you can buy sorbets or dairy-free ice creams. You can also encourage your child to start applying cream as young as possible so that it becomes as natural as cleaning his or her teeth. At first supervision will be needed, but the more your child can do for her- or himself the better.

Pets are another common source of eczema with children. If your child is allergic to dogs or cats it is obvious that you should avoid having pets, heartbreaking though this can be. It is also difficult if your child's friends or relatives have pets, and this can lead to family misunderstandings. People who do not understand about eczema can frequently be unsympathetic. Since the rash does not appear at once, they can also think that you are making an unnecessary fuss, as your child's eczema does not visibly worsen until they have left the house.

If you are reading this book because your new baby has just been diagnosed as suffering from eczema, do not despair. Most eczema is not very severe, and in the majority of cases a good skin-care regime and care with their diet can prevent the condition becoming a serious problem. In some cases, with proper care and treatment, the symptoms can be alleviated or even prevented entirely. Alternative or complementary therapies encourage the body's own natural healing process so they can offer a great deal of help for children and parents whose lives are affected by eczema.

The cure for eczema may therefore be well within your grasp. With any luck, after you have read this book, your child will be free from the symptoms of eczema; if not, at least you will be armed with knowledge to help you overcome it and, perhaps most of all, know that you and your child are not alone.

Note: 'He' and 'she' have been used to describe your child in alternate chapters to avoid the more cumbersome 'he or she'.

# Chapter One

# What is eczema?

Eczema is a condition of the skin which is now also known as dermatitis. It can vary from the very mild form, often known as a sensitive skin, in which the skin is often very dry, easily irritated and forms a rash, through a flaky, hot, itchy skin right through to the severe form in which the skin is broken, scaly, raw and bleeding, and can even become infected.

Eczema is closely linked to what is called contact dermatitis, when the skin produces a rash in response to some substance which irritates it. A large number of substances tend to irritate skin, and people with quite normal skins will often develop a rash in response to things like enzyme-containing detergents and some household or industrial chemicals. Nappy rash is very common, with the baby's skin flaring up as a result of contact with its urine and faeces, especially when they are left in contact for any length of time. Many people are allergic to some metals like nickel, which are used in cheap jewellery, metal buttons and zips. With most children who suffer from eczema, however, the cause or trigger of the rash is not obvious. The most common kind of eczema is known as atopic eczema (*see below*).

Eczema is not contagious, although the rash can be unsightly. In children, the main problem is skin irritation, which causes them to scratch and make the condition worse. While adults can usually stop themselves from scratching, young children are unable to restrain themselves. Children with eczema will therefore need special care to keep the condition under control.

There are different kinds of eczema, although all have similar, unpleasant symptoms. If you suspect your child has the condition you should always see a doctor, health professional or qualified alternative health practitioner for a proper diagnosis.

## CRADLE CAP

Cradle cap is a mass of thick, browny-yellow, greasy scales on top of the baby's head. It is very unsightly but normally does not itch or bother the baby. It almost always clears up on its own, usually by the age of two, and as the baby grows hair the condition often becomes less obvious. It can occasionally become infected if the infant, or more usually a parent who is bothered by the baby's appearance, scratches or picks at it.

## INFANTILE SEBORRHOEIC ECZEMA

This condition also appears on the scalp and looks very much like cradle cap. It may also appear first in the nappy area as a rash. Occasionally crusty patches of skin may also appear on the forehead, behind the ears, on the eyebrows, under the arm or on the trunk. It normally does not itch much or bother the child, and is usually outgrown quite quickly.

## ATOPIC (ALLERGIC) ECZEMA

The most common form of eczema is known as atopic eczema, and about 90 per cent of infants with eczema or dermatitis will be found to be atopic (the word comes from the Greek for 'alien', because the atopic person reacts to substances which are alien to it). This condition is closely linked to asthma, hay fever and other allergies, and these three conditions affect as many as 10 per cent of children.

The tendency to develop atopic eczema is largely inherited, so eczema, asthma and hay fever tend to run in families. If one parent is atopic the chance of having an affected child is doubled, and if both parents are affected the risk is increased fourfold. Atopic eczema is usually worse in childhood and tends to improve or even disappear as the child grows up.

Atopic eczema appears to be becoming more common, with as many as one in five children having some symptoms. Some people think that this is because of the increasing number of artificial chemicals in our environment, which either provoke a reaction themselves or combine with other common allergens. Artificial substances in the diet may also be more likely to provoke an allergic response.

People who are atopic tend to make larger than normal quantities of a specific type of antibody called immunoglobulin E (IgE for short). Antibodies exist to protect the body against foreign substances such as bacteria, viruses and various toxins. However, sometimes this reaction is provoked by a substance which is normally harmless and exists almost everywhere, such as pollen, dust particles, skin flakes from animals, especially cats (known as dander), and house-dust mites. Atopic people are also often more sensitive to chemicals found in household products such as soap, detergents, perfumes, bubble-baths and cleaning agents. With eczema, when the skin comes into contact with these substances it reacts, causing redness, itchiness and dryness of the skin.

Most babies are not born with eczema. It tends to emerge over the first year – 80 per cent of children who are going to develop eczema do so by their first birthday – but typically, babies are born with good skin. There may be other, early rashes which are common in all babies – *miliaria* or sweat rash, nappy rash, and cradle cap. Sometimes one of these early rashes seems to develop into atopic eczema, but more usually, the early rashes clear up and the eczema starts later, when the baby is two or three months old. The rash usually appears first on the cheeks, which may be red and dry-looking. As the baby starts to rub and scratch, the rash gets worse.

The first signs of atopic eczema in a young baby can also be restlessness and fretfulness and the baby tries to rub his head or back against the cot or pushchair, or tries to scratch. Red, weeping, crusted patches may appear on any part of the body, but in a young child the cheeks and the areas behind the ears are the most frequently affected. In toddlers the wrists and ankles are common sites, and in older children the eczema is often worst in the creases behind the knees and in the elbows.

Eczema does not always look the same on every child. Some children have very dry skin, and may have a rough, scaly kind of eczema (called ichthyosis, from the word meaning 'fish' in Greek, as the skin is dry and scaly). In some cases, the swollen blood vessels which make the skin look red can leak fluid, which causes the skin to swell and sometimes ooze, leading to fluid-filled blisters which then weep when scratched or rubbed. The fluid often contains clotting factors from the blood, so it causes crusts or scabs on the skin, which again the child tends to rub off. Excessive scratching can cause the skin to actually bleed. The condition sometimes appears in the form of rings on the skin, usually on the trunk. This rash looks very like ringworm and can be mistaken for it by parents, and even occasionally by health professionals.

Eczema may also cause changes in skin pigmentation, and this is particularly distressing for children with dark skin. It can interfere with the production of melanin in the skin, thus making it lighter. With very fair-skinned children this will not be noticeable, but in black children it can be more unsightly than the rash itself.

Frequent scratching can cause the skin to toughen, resulting in what is known as lichenification. In black children, this is often accompanied by an increase in black pigmentation, which can again look very unsightly. Some children have patches of lighter skin from scarring and darker skin where it has toughened and thickened. Fortunately this effect is not usually permanent and clears up when the eczema improves or is outgrown.

### ■ What happens to the skin in atopic eczema?

The skin is an important organ. It acts as a barrier between the body and the outside world, keeping harmful substances out and blood and fluids in. It also acts as a sense organ, containing receptors which convey sensations of heat and cold, texture, pain or pleasure to the brain, and helps to keep the body at a constant temperature. Some waste products are also eliminated through the skin via perspiration, and the skin helps manufacture vitamin D, which is made in response to sunlight on the skin and is needed by the body to help build up the bones and other tissues.

The skin is made up of two main layers: the outer or epidermis and the inner or dermis. The epidermis forms a tough, horny coating, and consists of dead skin cells which are constantly shed, to be replaced with new ones from the layer underneath. As the lower cells move towards the surface, they produce a protein called keratin which toughens them. Normally it takes about 28 days for a cell to be formed, move up to the surface, die off and be shed. This outer layer of skin largely prevents fluids from leaking out of the body or getting in.

The dermis is a thicker layer which contains the blood vessels and nerve fibres. The blood carries nutrients to the skin, and is also involved in the healing process when the skin is damaged or broken. Nerve fibres send signals to the brain about the environment in which it finds itself, and these help protect the skin itself and the whole body. Also found in the dermis are the sweat glands which cool the body down and are also activated by stress, and sebaceous (oil) glands which keep the skin moist and lubricated. Collagen and other fibres are found in the skin and give it its elasticity, which tends to diminish with age.

Because the skin is on the outside of the body it is particularly liable to damage, and this is particularly true in young children. The skin can be damaged by too much sunlight (causing sunburn), by cold (causing frostbite), by scratches, blows and other traumas, by chemicals, by insect bites and by infections.

The skin can also be damaged by processes occurring inside the body, which is what happens when you develop eczema.

The basic reaction of the skin in eczema is inflammation. The skin cells are stimulated by foreign substances, either on the skin or brought in through the blood supply, to produce substances called prostaglandins. These provoke the release of fluid into the tissues, causing them to swell, and the blood supply to the area increases, causing redness of the skin. Specialized white blood cells called lymphocytes rush to the area through the increased supply of blood and lymph, looking for the foreign substances to attack. The area becomes swollen, hot, red and sore.

Antibodies are produced to counter the foreign substance, which is known as an antigen or, in the case of a harmless substance which provokes an allergic response, an allergen. These antibodies stimulate the production of substances called histamines, which also provoke inflammation. The inflammation tends to weaken the horny, outer layer of skin. The child, irritated and sometimes driven to distraction by the soreness and itching, starts to scratch the skin, causing more damage to the outer layer. If the itching and scratching continue the outer layers become broken, and a raw, irritated, weeping skin results, which can sometimes lead to infection by bacteria. If the skin heals and forms a scab, this also tends to itch, and children will frequently scratch off the scab, leaving the skin open to infection again.

## ■ INFECTED ECZEMA

If the skin is broken, it is quite common for eczema to become infected with bacteria. Bacteria are found naturally on the skin and in the air, soil and water. Some bacteria normally live on the skin and these can often have a protective rather than harmful effect, producing substances which tend to repel other, often more harmful, bacteria. If the skin is damaged or broken, however, the more harmful bacteria, which are normally kept at bay or are present on the skin only in small quantities, may be able to multiply. These harmful bacteria tend to thrive in moist places and the scratched and broken skin of a child with eczema can provide a perfect breeding ground.

The most common bacterial infection of the skin is *Staphylococcus aureus*, which causes impetigo or boils. If this bacterium invades skin broken by eczema, it can cause a sudden worsening of the condition. The eczema will spread and become weepy, with yellow crusts and sometimes oozing pus. The child may have a slight temperature and the lymph nodes in the neck or groin may be swollen. Antibiotics may be needed to clear up the infection.

Although it is usually obvious when a child's eczema becomes infected with bacteria, this is not always the case. Since eczema tends to fluctuate in severity, and infected skin does not always lead to the above symptoms, parents may not realize that the skin is infected. You should always check that any sudden worsening of your child's eczema is not due to an infection.

A swab of the infected skin can be taken to find out which bacteria are responsible for the infection and what antibiotic it will be sensitive to. Unfortunately, the swab technique will only show whether the bacteria is present, not how many bacteria there are on the skin and therefore how serious a problem it is and whether it is really the bacteria which are causing a worsening of the eczema. Very occasionally the swabbing will reveal the presence of a more harmful strain of bacteria which should not normally be present on the skin at all, such as *Group A streptococcus*. This bacterium causes sore throats and is sometimes involved in rare heart and kidney infections, so a child who has it will need to be treated.

One problem with bacterial infections in eczema is that the bacteria tend to be passed around the family from the infected child to others. If this happens, the whole family need to take great care of hygiene, washing regularly, and the child with eczema needs to be kept scrupulously clean and the skin protected with oils and creams which tend to repel the bacteria.

## ▮ ECZEMA HERPETICUM

One rare complication of eczema is that the damaged skin can be infected by the cold-sore virus, *Herpes simplex*. This is one of the most common viruses and is very infectious, especially in children who do not have any immunity. Normally cold sores appear around the mouth, and are passed on by kissing. In most cases people become immune to the virus and cannot be infected again, although it can remain in the skin and be reactivated when the person is run down. However, if the virus gets into the bloodstream via the broken skin of someone with eczema it can be very serious; it can spread throughout the bloodstream and even affect the internal organs.

*Eczema herpeticum* normally appears on the skin in little clusters which look like small blisters. These are filled with a clear fluid at first, then produce pus. The blisters are scratched, become raw and weepy and start to have a crusted look. You should suspect *Eczema herpeticum* if the eczema seems to become worse and you can see the small blisters described above. It is usually accompanied by a high temperature and the affected person will feel very lethargic and unwell. You should seek medical advice immediately and mention your suspicions to the doctor, as it is a rare condition and can sometimes be missed. In extremely rare cases a child may die from this infection, so it is very important that you do not delay and seek help as soon as it is suspected.

Treatment is with the antiviral drug acyclovir. This can be given as an injection, by mouth or as an ointment, but it works most rapidly and effectively when it is given intravenously by drip in hospital. It can be given by mouth if the infection is caught in the early stages, otherwise a short stay in hospital is usually necessary.

Sometimes the infection recurs, though usually not as severely as the first time. It may therefore be sufficient to use the cream externally if you start early enough, and it should be applied five times a day for maximum effect. You should never attempt to

treat your child yourself, however, without seeking medical help
and obtaining a diagnosis.

### Case Study

Polly had very bad eczema which became infected with herpes
at one point, causing her to be rushed into hospital. Her
mother gives the following account: 'Polly's eczema started at
about six weeks old. She had bad cradle cap, and then the
eczema started to appear everywhere. By six months it was very
bad so we went to the doctor. He wanted to give steroids
straight away, but at the time there was a scare about steroid
side-effects, skin thinning and so on, so we thought we'd try
alternatives first. We used evening primrose oil, and we got
referred to the homoeopathic hospital. We used a cream and
some drops, but at that time Polly had a very severe allergic
reaction. She was very dehydrated and was taken into hospital.
We never found out what caused it.

'We then saw a dietitian at the hospital. She did patch tests
and found that if Polly got milk products on her skin she
reacted. We had a long period of eliminating foods from her
diet and found she was allergic to dairy products, cheese, and
wheat (gluten).

'When Polly was two and a half her eczema was infected
with a herpes virus. The speed at which it happened was
frightening; her arm swelled up and she was very ill. She was
rushed into hospital and was in intensive care and then in
isolation for a week. The drugs she was given worked very
quickly, however, and the problem has not happened again.

'Polly is now ten and completely free from eczema.'

# Chapter Two

# Causes and triggers of eczema

Eczema is first and foremost a genetic condition, in that the susceptibility to it is definitely inherited. However, it is normally triggered by substances outside the body which make contact with the skin, or by substances which are ingested through the diet.

The most common external substances are house-dust mites and their excrement, which are found in bedding, pillows, carpets and dust, and which thrive in centrally heated houses; hairs and skin cells from cats and dogs; perfumes and cleaning agents found in cosmetics; toiletries, soaps, shampoos and detergents; and chemicals such as pesticides, fertilizers, and cleaners. Metals used in buckles, buttons and cheap jewellery can also often cause an irritant response.

The most common allergens in the diet appear to be cow's milk and other dairy produce, tomatoes and citrus fruit, yeast containing foods, wheat, and a number of additives (*see* chapter 4). But there is a difference between allergy and food intolerance. An allergy is a direct response to an allergen, causing a skin rash, vomiting, or in extreme cases, anaphylactic shock (*see* page 16). Food intolerances are more difficult to detect, as the response is less obvious; a child's eczema may fluctutate and the rash may be difficult to pinpoint to a particular food eaten at a particular time.

**Food allergies and intolerances**

The term 'food allergy' is normally used when the child has a dramatic or obvious reaction to eating a food which occurs soon after touching or taking it – for instance, developing a rash around the mouth or more generally soon after taking the food, or being sick, or having a more severe response (see 'anaphylactic shock', page 16). The term 'food intolerance' is used when the reaction to a food is less clearcut and may occur some hours or even days after the food is taken, so is often masked. For a long time the medical establishment was fairly sceptical about food intolerances, but it is now accepted that these cause symptoms such as eczema and asthma, headaches and migraines, digestive problems, chronic fatigue and irritability.

Allergies and food intolerances may also be due to the increasing number of pollutants and chemicals in the air and in our diet. The average child's diet contains many pesticides, fungicides, dyes, and chemical preservatives. Moreover the modern diet, especially that of children, tends to be too high in sugars and refined carbohydrates, and too low in the vitamins and minerals necessary for building a healthy immune system.

## FINDING OUT WHAT YOUR CHILD IS ALLERGIC TO

Many parents find out what their children are allergic to simply through a process of trial and error. They notice that when they have certain foods, the eczema appears or flares up.

### Case Study

Dairy products were a problem for Maggie's baby Frank: 'Frank had been breastfed for six months, and the day after I gave him a cow's milk yoghurt for pudding these round, red, raised rings appeared all over his skin and back. Not knowing what it was, I took him to the doctor, who said it was eczema. I gave him goat's milk products for another month and he was fine. The next time I gave him food with milk in, the rash reappeared.

'For a long time I kept Frank off any cow's milk products. By the time he was two he could have small quantities of butter or cheese and by the time he was five it wasn't really a problem, as long as he didn't eat a wide range of dairy products every day.'

If you suspect a food allergy, it can help to have your child allergy tested. One such test is the patch test. This involves deliberately placing potential allergens onto an area of skin unaffected by the eczema, such as the back or an arm. Each patch is covered with a plaster for 24–48 hours and then the skin is examined. If there is a reaction, an allergy is suspected. However, these tests are not always completely reliable.

Another is the skin prick test. A solution is made up containing small quantities of the potential allergen, and this is introduced into the skin by pricking with a sterile needle. If the child is allergic to the substance, there will be a slightly raised lump or weal 15 minutes later. Because most children are afraid of pricks or needles, however, the patch test is usually preferred.

A third way of testing for allergies is through an elimination diet. It is important to do this under the guidance of your doctor or healthcare practitioner. The classic elimination diet requires fasting for four days, at its strictest taking only pure mineral water. Since this is not really feasible with children, the child is normally given three foodstuffs which almost never provoke an allergic response: lamb, pears and rice. Other foods are introduced one by one to see if they cause a reaction.

### Case Study

'When Callum was 14 months the eczema was really bad although I had cut out more and more foods – dairy, wheat, tomatoes, citrus fruit. The consultant suggested that if we [his parents] wanted to go down that route we should try a proper elimination diet. I was worried Callum wouldn't eat anything but he didn't seem to mind being given the same three foods every day at every meal. The consultant said that the diet wouldn't be easy and she also said that if this didn't work I would have to accept that it was more than diet which was causing the problem, which in the end it was.'

It is possible to check for allergies with a breast-fed child who is starting on solids. You should introduce each new food one at a time and gradually, so that any reactions can be put down to one specific food. David Atherton at Great Ormond Street Hospital in London suggests that a simple elimination diet may help up to 40 per cent of babies under one, up to 30 per cent of children between one and four and up to 20 per cent of those aged between 5 and 8. He also points out that care needs to be taken that the child is receiving nutritious alternatives. He believes that an adequate skin-care regime should always be tried first as the child's suffering through being denied foods is sometimes greater than that caused by the eczema.

It is important to realize that dietary restrictions can have a big impact on a child's social life, affecting their enjoyment of parties, social occasions and visits to friends, and that young children cannot understand why you are forbidding them foods that they like. Food is seen as symbolic of love, and the child is dependent on the mother to feed him or her, so denying food can be interpreted as withholding love and even the means of survival. Special diets should therefore be embarked on with care, and always with the help of a qualified person who can suggest alternatives to foods which are cut out and check that the child will be adequately nourished.

### Diagnosing atopic eczema

Blood tests can be carried out to diagnose atopic eczema, in which the number and types of white cells in the blood are measured. Someone with atopic eczema will often have an increased number of white cells called eosinophils. The blood test will also measure the level of immunoglobulin E (IgE) in the blood, which is usually raised. A more specialized test, the RAST test, can detect the existence of various types of IgE that are directed against specific allergens, such as cat hair, pollen or certain foods. Among the alternative therapies, there are other diagnostic techniques such as kinesiology and dowsing.

## Case Study

In their efforts to establish what Amy was allergic to, her parents tried kinesiology: 'The therapist tested for allergies by holding the potential allergic substances on her tummy. I held Amy's hand and held my other hand up, and when she was allergic to something I couldn't hold my hand up. It was very curious. The therapist discovered that she was allergic to a lot of foods including dairy products.'

## ■ THE ATOPIC CHILD

The child who has atopic eczema frequently suffers from other atopic conditions such as hay fever (rhinitis), asthma and allergies, sometimes resulting in hives (urticaria) or anaphylactic shock.

## Case Study

Joshua's mother spent the early years of his life dealing with the problems of having a highly allergic child. The first problem which emerged was eczema: 'Joshua always had very dry skin. As a small baby he had colic, and he kept getting nappy rash, although I changed his nappy all the time. Because he seemed very hungry he started on solids at three and a half months, and his eczema really started then. It was round his mouth, his joints and in the nappy area. He wore cotton clothes to keep him cool but covered up so he wouldn't scratch. It was difficult keeping the temperature constant, as he would easily get too cold or too hot. People said I was always fussing but I was trying to keep the eczema down.

'Between one year and 18 months it got very bad. I didn't want to keep going with the steroid cream we were prescribed so I tried homoeopathy. We cut out dairy products and gave him soya milk. Then when he was 18 months old we tried Chinese herbal medicine. Within three days the eczema had gone, it was like a miracle. We went back twice, but then Joshua had a massive asthma attack. At this point we had to seek conventional medical help.

'His eczema was up and down. We worked very hard on his skin. We bathed him twice a day, used special bath oil and lots of aqueous cream, and when it started to flare up badly we used steroid cream. But then his allergies started to emerge.

'The worst is sesame seed. After eating a bar with sesame in it Joshua went into anaphylactic shock and was rushed back into hospital just after he'd come out after an asthma attack. Then there is egg – if he gets egg anywhere on his skin he gets a rash, especially round his mouth, and he is sick if he eats any. He reacts to pollen with hay fever and asthma and he is allergic to talcum powder, tarnished metals, house-dust mites, concrete and plaster. If he comes into contact with these things he gets a skin rash, red with white bobbly spots, and then he scratches it and spreads it. We try to act quickly to wash it off rather than using antihistamines, which make him drowsy. We always have to bathe him after sports, and often when he's been to people's houses where there might be cats and dogs or lots of dust.

'We bought a non-allergic mattress. I boil-wash all his bedding constantly and damp-dust everything in the house. We have stripped wood floors and I keep all his toys in boxes so they don't collect dust. I have to be careful about which detergents and cleaning agents I buy, and I dry all his clothes indoors because of dust and pollen in the air.

'Until Joshua was six or seven he took an inhaled anti-allergy drug to prevent the asthma, but that stopped working, so now he has a mild dose of inhaled steroids. Because of this we don't want to use much steroid cream on his skin. The eczema is much better now he's ten but I still need to cream him regularly to keep his skin moist, and his allergies are still a problem.

'Having said all this, Joshua is an incredibly bouncy, energetic child with lots of friends and doing very well at school. He has developed a very sensible attitude to his allergies. He knows what he can and can't eat, and he knows what to do if he does have an allergic reaction – wash himself down thoroughly and take his antihistamines. We try not to restrict his activities and he leads a very normal life. His allergies have improved as he's got older and we can only hope he grows out of them entirely.'

## ■ ANAPHYLACTIC SHOCK

The atopic child with eczema may have a particularly severe reaction to an allergen. This is rare, but it can be a medical emergency. Anaphylactic reactions normally result from the injection of allergic substances into the blood – antibiotics and vaccine injections, and bee and wasp stings. It can also happen after eating some foods, and this is more common among children who have eczema. Foods which most commonly produce this reaction are peanuts and eggs, and sometimes fish, milk and other nuts.

At its most severe, anaphylactic shock will cause a child suddenly to become very sweaty, collapse and lose consciousness. More often there is dizziness, headache, tightness in the chest, swelling of the face and sometimes the throat, and difficulty in breathing. In extreme cases the child may need resuscitating, and can die. A large dose of an antihistamine helps, together with injections of adrenalin. If your child has had a severe reaction to a drug, insect sting or food then you will probably be given an emergency injection to administer yourself.

Fortunately these reactions tend to become less severe as the child gets older, and most children will grow out of this kind of reaction completely. In the meantime, it is sensible to make sure that your child has the necessary drugs with her when she goes to school or visit friends and that they are told to call in medical help in case of an emergency.

Parents who have an atopic child can help prevent anaphylactic reactions by avoiding substances which are classic triggers such as nuts, especially peanuts. Read the labels on biscuits, cakes and other confectionary; increasingly attention is being drawn to the presence of nuts in foods. Some creams and oils used in cosmetics can also contain nuts. For example peanut oil was used in one kind of nipple cream until recently, and could be ingested by a breast-feeding baby, so check any products which you use on your or your baby's skin.

# Chapter Three

# Helping your child

The old adage that prevention is better than cure is certainly true when it comes to eczema. Caring for the skin, watching the diet, wearing appropriate clothing and keeping the environment free of allergens, can prevent eczema becoming a problem. In addition, reducing the exposure to allergens can enable your child's body to re-balance and encourage the body's own natural healing process.

One of the most difficult aspects of treating eczema is that it seems to come and go, getting worse and then improving, sometimes for no obvious reason. If it is linked to specific allergens, it may become worse in the spring when there is pollen, or in the winter when your child spends more time indoors. Sunshine and fresh air may help, or it may make it worse. Stress and the mental state of both the child and the parents can also affect eczema, so it is not always clear which treatment is working and which is not.

Another important fact to remember is that almost all children grow out of eczema. In fact, it is most common among very young children. If a child is going to develop eczema, it is very likely that it will appear in the first year of life. Forty per cent of children who develop eczema do so by three months, 65 per cent by six months and 80 per cent by one year. It may then take some years for it to reach its worst, but then it usually starts to improve again. The eczema will come back and go away, but the typical pattern is for it to improve first only for a short time, and then for longer and longer periods, until the skin is clear more often than it is bad. Most people who have had bad eczema in childhood will continue to have a sensitive skin, which may flare up from time to time, perhaps in periods of intense stress or when the skin has come into contact with some irritant. But it will no longer dominate their life as it did in the past.

Of those children who developed eczema by one year, about 50 per cent will stop having a problem by the age of five. Only 25 per cent will still be having problems by the age of nine, 12 per cent by 13, 6 per cent by 17, and 3 per cent by the age of 21. For those people whose eczema starts later, however, the chances of it lasting longer are increased.

## PREVENTING ECZEMA

There are measures you can take to try to prevent your child developing eczema, or, if the eczema has emerged, to keep it at bay. These involve diet (which will be discussed in the next chapter), household cleanliness, and avoiding irritant substances.

### Avoiding allergens in the home

It can be very important to keep the child's environment as clean as possible and free from dust, which often harbours the house-dust mite. The dust mites, known by the horrible-sounding names *Dermatophagoides pteronyssimus* and *Dermatophagoides farinae*, live mainly off the flakes of dead skin which form a large part of ordinary household dust. The tiny creatures are invisible to the naked eye but thrive in warm, centrally heated houses, being found in mattresses, duvets and blankets, pillows, carpets, cushions, soft furnishings and children's cuddly toys. It is mainly the droppings which cause the allergy or intolerance. Children whose skin is already damaged with eczema will be more vulnerable as the mite products may be scratched into already sensitive skin. The tiny faecal particles can also cause sneezing, hay fever or asthma if inhaled.

If your child has eczema it is important to keep surfaces wiped clean and rooms free of dust. Damp-dusting is best, so that the allergens are not spread around the room. Regular vacuuming under the bed and in corners is important. If you can, have a wooden or vinyl floor which can be kept clean and dust-free, perhaps with rugs which can be removed regularly for cleaning. Your child's mattress should be vacuumed regularly and the bedding washed. You can also buy special covers for mattresses, pillows and duvets. You need to wash bedding at a temperature of at least 60 degrees to kill house-dust mites, but if this is not possible, duvets, blankets and pillows can be put in the freezer overnight before or after washing to kill them off. Cuddly toys, especially when kept in your child's bed, should be subjected to the same treatment. Feathers and natural fibres tend to attract house-dust mites more than artificial ones, so it can help to have man-made fibres in pillows and duvets, and have a carpet that contains little or no wool. Try to have enough cupboards and toy chests for most objects to be put away where they will not collect dust. The whole house should be damp-dusted regularly and curtains and carpets regularly cleaned. An ioniser can be used to precipitate dust from the air.

Some common moulds and fungi can also be allergens for the atopic child, especially *Cladiosporum herbarum* and *Alternaria alternata*. These are found in rooms with rising damp or where there is excessive condensation. They can also live on some foods, including apples, dried fruit and some beans and grains. It is obviously important to keep your home well heated and well ventilated if this is at all possible, and if not, to move or apply to be rehoused if your child's health is suffering.

Recent research has shown that another common fungus, *Pityrosporum ovale*, a yeast fungus which is present on everyone's skin, may be important in atopic eczema. It is now thought to aggravate the condition in a proportion of people, especially those with a pattern of severe eczema on the head and torso.

Treatment with antifungal medicine can produce a good improvement.

## *Pets*

Pets can be a problem for an allergic child. Animal fur and shed skin are frequent allergens. Cats in particular are likely to cause a problem, as they shed flakes of skin or dander continuously, and their saliva and urine are also allergenic. Some children are so sensitive to cats that they will react to a room in which a cat has been one or two days previously. Others may be able to stroke a cat without any reaction, but it is a different matter to have a cat living in a house.

If your child is desperate for a pet, it may be better to have something like a rabbit or guinea pig which can live out of doors and to which the child's exposure is limited. If you already have a dog or cat, it can be heartbreaking for your child to part with it, but if his reaction is severe giving the animal to a caring relative or friend may be the only solution. If your child reacts to animals it can also be important to make sure visitors do not bring animals to the house.

It can take some weeks or even longer for the eczema to clear up after you have parted with a pet, as it may take that long for the last traces of dander to be removed from the furnishings, carpets and so on.

## Clothing

It is very important that your child wears light, loose-fitting clothes made from natural fibres which allow the skin to breathe and keep him cool. If the skin overheats and perspiration is left to dry on it, your child will start to itch and then scratch, and a vicious circle is started up.

With babies and young children clothes are not much of a problem. Cotton baby suits are readily available, and some have built-in mittens which will help stop them from scratching. You can also buy scratch mittens, although these tend to work loose. Cotton sheets, light bedding and cotton air blankets are also available and will allow your baby's skin to breathe.

For older children, cotton clothes may be more expensive, but they are generally available. Loose cotton T-shirts and sweatshirts and cotton jogging trousers are often the most comfortable. Leather shoes with leather soles are best, and it is a good idea to avoid the excessive use of trainers or shoes which have a soft, spongy artificial lining, as these tend to make the feet hot and sweaty. Cotton socks are also a must. Avoid wool, which is itchy, and polyester, which does not breathe.

By the time your child is of school age, clothing can become a real problem. Many schools have school uniforms which are often made from synthetic fibres, and these are popular with parents because they are cheap and hard-wearing, and because they do not need ironing. However they are a recipe for disaster for a child with eczema.

Fortunately there are alternatives. Often cotton clothes can be found. If not you may need to have some made or ask the school to allow cotton trousers or a jacket that it non-regulation as long as it is in a similar style and colour.

## Skin care

Perhaps the most important thing any parent can do to prevent eczema is care for the skin. This means keeping it clean, moisturized, and avoiding soaps, bubble baths and other products which dry and irritate the skin. A baby with sensitive skin will need more frequent bathing than most to keep the skin clean. A young baby should be washed in warm water, without soaps or bubble-baths. A little baby oil or emollient in the bathwater will help keep the skin moist.

Babies with eczema will also need to wear loose, comfortable cotton clothing and will probably need to have their nappies changed more often than usual. Some parents find that their baby's skin reacts to the bleaches or other chemicals in disposable nappies, so it is worth trying a number of brands. Some mothers find that terry nappies are best, especially when washed in non-biological detergents. Others find that disposable nappies keep their baby's skin drier and more comfortable.

It is best to avoid detergents with enzymes, perfumes or colourings, and you may find that fabric softeners irritate your baby's skin. There are some detergents available which are advertised as 'for sensitive skin'.

*Topical applications*

Topical treatments are those that are applied directly to the skin. The most important treatments for eczema are the variety of creams, oils and ointments which are designed to keep the skin moist. There are creams and ointments with other added ingredients such as herbs and plant oils which are often beneficial, but here we are concerned with the creams and ointments which are simply designed to moisten the skin.

Creams, ointments and lotions are actually different, although the terms are often used interchangeably. Ointments generally contain oil alone, almost always a mineral oil of a greasy consistency, usually white soft paraffin (like Vaseline), although other oils are added to give a slightly different 'feel'.

Creams consist mainly of water, to which oil has been added. As oil and water do not mix, an emulsifier is added to make the oil break into tiny droplets which are spread evenly through the water base. Lotions are just very watery creams, and oily creams are ointments to which water has been added.

Gels consist of water in which some other substance forms a lattice to provide a structure. Bath oils are oils which are designed to be used in the bath or shower. Some spread over the surface of the water so that they coat the skin as the child gets in or out of the bath, and others disperse in the water.

Almost all creams and ointments also contain preservatives to help cut down the growth of bacteria in them, and antioxidants to stop them breaking down, as butter does when it goes rancid.

Emulsifiers are used to stabilize the creams or ointments; one of the most common is lanolin, which is derived from sheep's wool and gives the cream a pleasant soft feel. Sometimes a fragrance is added.

Some moisturizers contain other ingredients which are intended to improve their moisturizing properties. These include lactic acid and urea. Lactic acid tends to be used where the skin is dry rather than open, cracked and weeping, as it can be irritating in severe eczema. Urea is a natural substance which is actually a waste product of body processes, and is found in large quantities in urine. It is able to penetrate the skin rapidly and it attracts water, thus helping to moisturize the skin.

One of the main problems with moisturizers is that they tend to provide a good breeding ground for bacteria, which can be introduced by unclean fingers. They multiply in the tub of cream, and can then be transferred in great numbers onto your child's skin, making it flare up and causing the eczema to become infected. Because of this, it is important to make sure that you wash your hands before dipping your fingers into the tub, and that your child does the same. It is less easy to introduce bacteria into tubes than tubs, so they are preferable when your child has to take cream or ointments into school or on day trips.

A small number of children with eczema will develop an allergy to the emulsifiers, preservatives, antioxidants or fragrances in creams or ointments. They therefore tend not to be effective, and may even occasionally make the child worse. Changing to a different kind of cream or ointment may make a difference.

The oilier preparations can occasionally make the skin too greasy, causing blackheads and other spots. This becomes particularly problematic when your child becomes an adolescent and the skin becomes greasier. It is best if this happens to change to one of the more watery creams.

The rule with all moisturizing creams and ointments is to use them little and often. Too much will waste the (sometimes expensive) product and make the skin too oily, and will get onto clothes, furnishings etc. Ideally they should be applied two to three times a day, in the morning, in the middle of the day and at night, although when the eczema is bad they can also be applied in between.

### Bathing
Moisturizers are at their most effective when used in the bath or shower. This is because the dry skin usually associated with eczema absorbs some of the water from the bath and can then be kept in by the layer of moisturizer.

Some people mistakenly think that you should not bath a child with eczema too often. In fact this is not the case. Bathing is vital in caring for the skin, but soap, bubble-baths and other cleansing agents should never be used on a child with eczema, as these tend to dry the skin. Bathing cleans the skin and helps prevent infection. The scales, crusts, dry skin, dirt and dried blood which accumulate on the skin and tend to attract bacteria can all be washed off, reducing the likelihood of infection. The skin is moisturized, and clean, softened, moisturized skin forms a better base for any other treatment which may be given.

Moreover, small children usually love their bath, and this can be a time for the child with eczema and the parent to enjoy a special time together. Putting on the creams can be fun, as well as being a gentle way of cleaning the skin.

Most eczema can be prevented or improved dramatically if the skin is kept soft and moist with regular applications of aqueous cream. This can be used two to three times a day as a preventive or treatment, being applied to the skin at least twice a day, in the morning and in the evening after the wash or bath. As soon as a patch of skin becomes inflamed it can be used during the day as well.

### Other skin remedies
If your child has a flare-up of eczema, putting two tablespoons of sodium bicarbonate in the bathwater can ease the itching. Calamine lotion is also very soothing, and can be dabbed on with cotton wool.

Nappy-rash ointment containing zinc oxide and cod liver oil is useful for nappy rash and eczema alike. For cradle cap, you can use olive oil rubbed into the scalp followed by a gentle shampoo, or there are special shampoos available for this condition.

## Psychological factors

It is known that eczema does have a psychological component. It can flare up, especially in teenagers and young adults, under the stress of examinations, family problems, a death or divorce, moving house or upsets in relationships. This emotional component may in fact go back to early childhood. The well-known psychotherapist Dinora Pines, who started life as a medical doctor and dermatologist, has written about this in her book, *A Woman's Unconscious Use of Her Body*. She writes that the skin is the main means of communication between mother and baby, and that skin-to-skin contact is intensely soothing for the newborn baby. 'The skin becomes a medium for physical contact, for the comfort of holding and being held . . . It is one of the most primitive channels for non-verbal communication.' When the infant's skin is damaged by a skin disorder, this will affect the amount of holding that goes on and may also affect the mother's relationship with the child. The child's demands may exceed that which the good-enough mother is able to provide. 'These babies not only suffer the physical discomfort of a damaged skin . . . they are also deprived of an adequate maternal mirroring response of admiration and love for the child's body.' She argues that this causes problems for the child which are often carried through into adult life.

Of course mothers whose babies have eczema can overcome these problems. But there is no doubt that in most cases, severe eczema will have an effect on both the mother and the child, as well as other family members, and this will also affect the relationship between them.

Bryan Lask, consultant psychiatrist at Great Ormond Street Hospital in London, believes that about 40 per cent of children with eczema have some psychological difficulties over and above the skin disorder. In his book *Atopic Eczema*, written for the British Society for Paediatric Dermatology, Mr Lask states:

> There is a complex interaction between emotional arousal and eczema. Emotional arousal leads to perspiration and increased sweating, which intensifies the eczema, which in itself becomes upsetting and distressing, perpetuating a vicious circle.

Some children undoubtedly do react strongly, blushing easily, readily becoming upset and finding it hard to face certain situations. This is especially true when a child suffers from a skin condition which may make him or her more than usually self-conscious.

### Case Study

Fiona's mother recalls the difficulties her daughter used to face at school. 'Appearing in any school performance or at a school assembly, or going into a room of new people, used to instantly make Fiona's eczema flare up. She would get agitated beforehand, go very quiet, and her skin would sometimes go bright red as if she was blushing all over her body, and then she would start itching. It was painful just to watch her.'

If your child's eczema is causing severe difficulties with regard to social life or relationships with others, he or she may benefit from counselling or therapy (*see* page 71).

*Helping your child's self-esteem*

A child with eczema can suffer from a loss of self-esteem, which can be as damaging and sometimes more lasting than the eczema itself. Our society is very much concerned with outward appearances, and children can suffer a great deal in social situations from stares, teasing and ill-considered remarks about their skin.

Although its obviously upsetting to have a child who is disfigured by a rash, it is important to praise your child and say how beautiful he is to you. As children grow older, you can continue to encourage them, praising the way they look and finding positive things to say about their appearance. You can also talk about the things other people say, helping your child to find ways of dealing with comments such as 'What's wrong with your skin?' or 'Is it catching?'

Children are also very quick to pick up on your own attitudes and feelings, and will often also overhear and understand what you say to other adults. Be careful not to talk about how awful your child looks when you are within earshot, and try not to talk continually about medicines, treatments and so on when he is present.

Praising your child in other ways can also help. If you have a healthy, positive attitude to eczema, he will copy you, to the benefit of both of you and, indeed, of the entire family.

### Helping other children in the family

Children who have eczema often receive more attention than others. The soothing of the skin with ointments and frequent bathing, feeding and picking up may mean that they receive more mothering. In fact, the condition can sometimes affect other children in the family more than the child with eczema. Siblings may feel that the other child is 'special', receiving special foods, special visits to the doctor or hospital, special soaps and special clothes. They may not realize that you are frantically trying to compensate for the fact that your child is missing out on other things.

Children are always looking out for signs that one of them is receiving more love and attention from the parents than the others, and it can be a very difficult balancing act for parents. It helps if you try to treat all the other children in the family in the same way. Rather than having special foods, try giving all the family the same diet as the child with eczema, or at least putting a substitute food available for everyone to try without drawing attention to it. Buy soaps which everyone can use and use special oils and creams on everyone's skin – they will all benefit from a little. If the child with eczema needs frequent bathing, it will do no harm for the other children to have a quick splash as well. Moisturizing creams will help all skins, and all the family will benefit from a dust-free house and the frequent washing of bedclothes.

Some children learn to use their eczema to manipulate their parents. 'If you don't let me do that I'll scratch' is one frequently used ploy. Once a child is old enough to understand that scratching will make the itch worse, they will soon realize that this strategy hurts only themselves, so long as the parents do not give in to it.

Giving your child responsibility for treating his or her own eczema as soon as possible can also help with siblings and with friends, as well as giving him or her more independence. The sooner children learn to bath themselves and rub cream on their own skin the easier it is for them to stay over at friends' houses, and the less their brothers and sisters feel they are being fussed over.

### Travel and holidays

Family holidays can become a nightmare when a child suffers from severe eczema. Heat, sun, wind, sea and sand can all combine to make the skin itchier than ever. It may be difficult to keep to a diet, new foods may aggravate the eczema, it may be difficult to bath or shower adequately or to wash clothes or find the right soaps and detergents. If the place you are staying in is not clean your child may be liable to infections.

Hot, sticky nights can make the normal itching from eczema seem intolerable and the whole family may go short of sleep. If the eczema becomes infected, or you run out of ointments or creams, there is the problem of how to find a doctor and explain what is wrong.

However, a holiday can be essential for the parents and the whole family, and there are ways around the problems with a little care and attention. Self-catering holidays are often best.

Some people find that holiday apartments with tiled floors and little furniture actually cause an improvement in their child's eczema, as do fresh sea air and sunshine. You can take your own bedding to make sure that it is not allergenic, and your own washing powder too. With self-catering it is also easier to control the child's diet.

You do have to be careful about your child's skin in the sun on holiday. While the sun can help – often after initially making the eczema worse for a few days – sunburn will not, and the combination of burned and eczematous skin can be sheer hell. It is important to limit your child's exposure to sunshine to 20 minutes in the heat of the day, and use a sun-block of at least factor 15 and preferably factor 25 once the skin has had its 20-minute dose. Most creams now block against both long- and short-wave ultraviolet rays, known as UVA and UVB, but read the label carefully, as creams which only block out UVB are not as good. You should always reapply the sunscreen after swimming, even if it says it is water-resistant, and at intervals throughout the day.

Sun hats and umbrellas are also a must. Remember too to pack your creams, emollients, special treats, plenty of cotton clothing, and medicines in case they are necessary.

### Organized holidays

It may also be possible for your child to go on holiday with a group. For example, the National Eczema Society in the UK, in conjunction with the National Asthma Campaign, organizes holidays for children who suffer from severe eczema. These can often be a boon for parents who need a break and for children who find that their needs are not usually understood. These holidays are for young people of different ages who have eczema and asthma, and they enable them to take part in a number of adventurous pursuits such as canoeing, wind-surfing, archery, climbing, cycling and ice skating. The idea is to bring together young people with similar problems in a safe environment, build their confidence and social skills, and enable them to enjoy themselves without fear that they will make their condition worse.

Each holiday group is closely supervised by a leader with a group of helpers, many of whom will have had first-hand experience of eczema. There are also nurses and a doctor who give the young people talks on how to manage their condition and are on hand to help if the eczema gets worse. Although the main emphasis is on having fun and trying out new activities, the idea is also that the children should get to know others in the same situation and talk openly and sympathetically to one another about their problems and treatments.

Information about these holidays can be obtained through the National Eczema Society (*see* 'Useful addresses' at the end of the book).

## HELP FOR PARENTS

Sometimes your child's eczema can seem to take over your whole life. The demands of the condition can create problems within a marriage, driving a wedge between father and mother. Some parents end up sleeping in different rooms, taking it in turns to care for the sleepless child. Lack of sleep makes both partners irritable and more prone to arguments. Since the mother is usually the prime carer, taking care of the child all day and then doing the lion's share of the nights because her partner has to go to work, it is often she who bears the brunt, feeling restricted in her activities. Some mothers delay returning to work because they are afraid no one else will take adequate care of their children or put up with their demands.

It is best to try not to let your child's eczema change your life. You should be able to find adequate child care or a nursery place, where your child's needs can be catered for, and a break from the problem may be the best thing for everyone. If at all possible, also try to find someone who can care for your child for a few hours while you and your partner go out together. If you are a single parent, and therefore bear the whole burden, try to make arrangements to have some time when you can go out and enjoy a few hours away from your child. Everybody needs a break some time, and for the parents of a child with eczema it can be vital.

There are many therapies and treatments available which can help you to deal with the stress of caring for your child. Yoga, relaxation and other classes are often available locally at very little cost. There are also therapies such as flotation, in which you are immersed in a warm bath of salty water, the lights are turned down and you drift away, listening to music or not as you prefer, in a deeply relaxing back-to-the-womb type experience. Aromatherapy massage, visualization, hypnosis and meditation can also help to relieve stress and enable you to cope better. Find out which works best for you and treat yourself whenever you can – you and your family will reap the benefits.

# Chapter Four

# Diet

## ▓ BREAST-FEEDING

Since cow's milk is a common trigger for eczema, it can be important to avoid it for as long as possible. For most mothers, this means breast-feeding if it is at all possible. If you or your partner suffer from eczema and you know your child is at increased risk, breast-feeding exclusively for the first four months and avoiding cow's milk products when she is weaned does seem to cut down the risk of eczema. If your first baby suffered from eczema, and especially if this developed after weaning from the breast, you might like to breast-feed your second child for longer. If the baby is going to react to cow's milk, the earlier it is introduced the more likely it is to trigger the allergy. So the longer you breast-feed your baby, the better the protective effect.

Most formula milks contain skimmed cow's milk or whey, with added vegetable fats. There are alternatives, such as soya-based milks, but in fact infants are as likely to react to these as to cow's milk, so they should only be tried once a cow's milk allergy has definitely been established. Some soya-based formulas have recently been shown to be high in aluminium levels, so they should really only be given after consultation with a health professional.

Breast-feeding does without doubt protect against atopic eczema, as well as asthma and hay fever. A report published in the medical journal *The Lancet* in 1995 followed up three groups of babies: those who were breast-fed for six months or more, for one to six months and for less than a month. They found that eczema at one and three years was lowest in the prolonged breast-feeding group. At the age of 17 only 8 per cent of the long-term breast-fed group had substantial atopy, compared with 23 per cent in the middle group and 54 per cent in the group who received little or no breast-feeding.

Unfortunately for mothers who choose to breast-feed, the practice of giving babies formula milk during the first days of life, while they are in hospital, is still too frequent. Even one bottle of formula milk given early by a nurse or midwife can sensitize the child to cow's milk. Sometimes a bottle is given because the mother is 'worn out' after labour and 'needs a rest'. Sometimes it is because the baby does not take the breast initially and concern about low blood sugar levels leads them to feel that the baby must be fed immediately. Giving a bottle is more common after a long labour or when the mother has had a Caesarean. So if you want to breast-feed in order to protect your child from atopic conditions, it is important to stress to hospital staff that you do not want any formula given unless this is absolutely necessary and you have discussed it with a paediatrician and consented.

### The mother's diet

Another issue is the mother's diet when breast-feeding. It has been shown that antigens produced by the mother in response to foods she eats can pass through into the breast milk. Intact cow's milk proteins may pass through into the breast milk, and sensitize the baby, although the effect may only become apparent later on when the child is weaned and given cow's milk products.

A mother who had severe eczema herself and perhaps whose partner had eczema, and who therefore knows that her baby is at high risk, might like to avoid wheat, eggs and cow's milk proteins while breast-feeding. It is also important that you eat alternative sources of calcium and first-class protein. The easiest way is to eat more meat and fish. If you are a vegetarian it would be best to seek the advice of a dietitian. Indeed, if you are cutting out any major part of your diet it is best to discuss it first with a dietitian or health practitioner.

### Breast-feeding and the immune system

Breast-feeding is also known to help boost the infant's immune system. The colostrum, the yellowish fluid produced in the first few days after the baby is born, contains high levels of antibodies, including one called secretory IgA, which is thought to help line the intestines, preventing foreign substances from passing through the infant's rather 'leaky' gut wall. Human milk contains a large number of enzymes and also white blood cells, which can attack bacteria, fungi and intestinal parasites. Human milk also contains lactoferrin, which inhibits the growth of bacteria and fungi in the gut; cow's milk by contrast encourages the growth of the bacteria needed to help digest grass. Breast-fed babies develop a healthy intestinal flora which helps them avoid digestive problems and resist gastro-intestinal infections.

If mother and baby are exposed to infection, the mother immediately starts producing antibodies to that specific bacterium or virus, and these antibodies are passed on to the baby in the milk, to help the new infant resist the infection. Not surprisingly, studies have repeatedly shown that breast-fed babies are less liable to infections, especially the respiratory infections and gastro-intestinal infections which can threaten a new baby's health and life.

### Help and support for mothers

Most mothers want the best for their baby and know that breast-feeding is best. Unfortunately this knowledge means that many women who do not breast-feed or who give up early feel that they are failures. Given the necessary help and support, the majority of women can succeed in breast-feeding, and most babies are capable of feeding at the breast, but it is a skill which has to be learned, and in our society far too few mothers get the help and support they need. They can encounter severe difficulties, including problems in getting the baby correctly latched on, sore nipples (which usually occur when the baby is not latched on well), blocked ducts and mastitis. Others have very unsettled babies who cry and feed more than average and always appear hungry. Others may need to go back to work or have other commitments which make extended breast-feeding difficult or impossible. There is no point in making yourself feel guilty if circumstances mean that you cannot continue breast-feeding or need to wean your child from the breast.

Advice and support for breast-feeding is available. In the UK, for example, there is a national network of breast-feeding counsellors trained by the National Childbirth Trust, and a new organization called the Breast-feeding Network. These are volunteers who have all breast-fed their own babies and who can provide information about breast-feeding and counsel you if you have difficulties. The La Leche League also has trained breast-feeding supporters. The addresses of two of these organizations are given under 'Useful addresses' at the end of the book.

## WEANING AND FIRST FOODS

Babies should be on a diet of breast milk or formula milk alone for the first four to six months of their life. At four months the first solids can be introduced, and you need to give foods that are unlikely to provoke allergies such as stewed fruit (pears, apples, apricots), rice and some vegetables. Cereals like rice and oats are preferable to wheat (prepared foods will have the label 'gluten free'). Tomatoes, strawberries and nuts should be avoided.

Once your baby starts to be weaned she will still need milk. All babies under six months of age must have breast milk or modified cow's milk (formula). After six months you can continue to give breast milk or formula, or you can use goat's milk or soya milks. The longer you stay off cow's milk products the less likely they are to be a problem, and the same applies to other potential allergens.

Goat's milk is in fact more similar to human milk than cow's milk, but it is still unmodified and should never be given to a baby under six months. Some goat's milks are unpasteurized and should not be given to young children because of the risk of bacterial infection in a baby whose immune system is still not fully developed. If you do give unpasteurized goat's milk to a child under one it should be boiled first.

Ready-to-drink soya milks, as opposed to soya formulas, do not contain enough calcium, so if your baby is only having soya milk you should make sure she gets additional sources of calcium.

You can cut out the obvious sources of cow's milk such as milk, yoghurt, ice cream, cheese and butter, but it is not always realized that many margarines contain skimmed cow's milk or whey, or that many biscuits, soups, and pre-packed meals contain milk products. You can get a list from a dietitian about safe foods but going on an entirely milk-free diet may mean buying food in Jewish supermarkets, health-food shops and other specialist outlets.

## A HEALTHY DIET

The increasing numbers of pesticides, fungicides, preservatives, sweeteners, flavourings, colourings and other additives in food may be a factor in the increasing number of food allergies. These artificial chemicals may combine with the natural foodstuffs to produce an allergic response. It goes without saying that your child will be less likely to develop allergic conditions if she eats a healthy diet, with fresh fruit, raw or lightly cooked vegetables, and freshly prepared foods. Organic meat, organic milk and dairy products and organic vegetables are increasingly available.

Studies have shown that today's children tend to eat far too many processed foods, with a diet high in crisps, chips, fried foods such as cheap burgers, and sweetened and salted baked beans or other convenience foods. Many children prefer white, steamed bread to wholemeal alternatives, and many popular breakfast cereals have a high sugar content. Children also consume large quantities of biscuits, chocolate bars, sweets and fizzy sweet drinks.

**Foods for older children and teenagers**
Older school-age children and teenagers often become very fussy about their diet, and are often influenced by their peers and the 'in' foods advertised on television. It can help if you cook healthier versions of popular foods such as burgers and pizzas. Many teenagers become concerned about animal welfare and the environment, and their idealism can be harnessed to help them to understand why it is important to eat healthy foods such as organic meat and milk and vegetables, as this also benefits animals. Concern about keeping slim can also be used to help teach teenage children the importance of a healthy diet. If your child has eczema, you can also explain about the importance of diet in keeping eczema under control, especially if it is linked to food intolerances.

Many processed, frozen and ready-made meals have been cooked for long periods, which removes many of the vitamins necessary for healthy skin. Vitamin B3 (nicotinic acid or niacin and nicotinamide), for example, is an essential vitamin; a shortage of it causes pellagra, which is characterized by dermatitis as well as, in extreme cases, diarrhoea and dementia. Vitamin B3 is found in beef, milk, fish and whole grains, though maize flour is short of it. A shortage of vitamin B2 (riboflavin) and B6 (pyridoxine) causes a red, greasy, scaly facial skin. Vitamin B2 is found in meats, milk, cereal and some green, leafy vegetables, and vitamin B6 is found in most meats, fish, egg yolk, wholegrain cereals, bananas, avocados, nuts, seeds and some leafy green vegetables.

## Food additives

Children with eczema should whenever possible be given fresh foods. Convenience foods should be as free as possible from additives, preservatives, colourings and flavourings, as these may provoke an allergic reaction in a sensitive child.

Food additives will be listed on food labels as E numbers. Not all of them are harmful: E160, for instance, is carotene, a naturally occurring colouring found in carrots. The groups of additives which are believed to aggravate eczema particularly are the azo dyes and the benzoate preservatives. There are 11 azo dyes, the most common of which are tartrazine (E102), sunset yellow (E110), amaranth (E123) – a red dye – and ponceau 4R (E124), which is green. Others are E107, E122, E128, E180, E151, E154 and E155. There are ten benzoate preservatives with numbers E210 to E219.

## Helping your child lead a normal life

It is important to resist the temptation to be overprotective. You should allow your child to do what other children do as much as possible. Changes in diet can have important consequences for the child, as food in our culture is symbolic of others things. It is seen by children as a way in which parents show their love. If you withhold treats or foods your child likes, she may think you are withholding love. Similarly, if your child has food which is different from other children, this can create social difficulties. If a would-be friend offers your child a chocolate and she refuses it, the other child will feel rebuffed, not understanding that your child cannot eat it. It is important not to let food restrictions become an ordeal for your child during social occasions, school meals, visiting friends or going to parties.

### Case Study
It is probably best to waive the normal rules occasionally, as with children's parties. 'We used to send Darren to parties with

a little box of his own "safe" foods,' recalls Sally. 'It was only when I went to a party early and saw him standing on his own in a corner nibbling at a sandwich while everyone else was sitting round the table eating crisps and chocolate cake that I realized he was missing out socially. We would make an extra effort to put cream on his skin and be aware that his eczema would be bad for a few days afterwards, but it seemed better to let him be like the others sometimes. When he got older he would learn to sit up with the others and just eat a small quantity of "forbidden" foods without drawing attention to himself and to the fact that he was "different".'

# Chapter Five

# Conventional treatments

Conventional treatment for eczema consists mainly of skin-care medications which contain steroids. Many doctors will combine these with the emollient creams and lotions and moisturizers described in chapter 3. Parents may however hesitate to use steroid treatments on their child's skin because of the risk of side-effects (*see* pages 42–4), and there are many other remedies available (*see* chapter 6). However, in some cases the eczema is so severe, the child is so miserable and the skin is so damaged that steroid creams may be necessary to break the cycle of itching and scratching, allow the skin to heal and stop the damage from worsening. In some cases the raw skin becomes infected and this too may need medical treatment.

## ▦ STEROIDS

Corticosteroid drugs (often just called steroids), in the form of creams and ointments, are the most common treatment for eczema. They are known as topical steroids – because they are applied to the skin – to distinguish them from steroids which are taken internally.

Steroids are a group of natural hormones produced in the body by a variety of different glands including the pituitary, thyroid, adrenal glands and the pancreas. The outer layer or cortex of the adrenal glands produces corticosteroids. Some of these affect the reproductive system, and others the salt and water balance of the body. A third group, known as glucocorticoids, act to cut down inflammation and suppress certain immune responses. Because of their effects these drugs, the most important of which is cortisol (usually called hydrocortisone in its manufactured form), were hailed as wonder drugs when they were first discovered. Those used in the treatment of eczema today are mainly synthetic drugs which are more powerful and thus more effective, such as prednisolone and prednisone, which are usually given by mouth, and betamethasone, fluocinolone, and clobetasone, which are usually applied to the skin.

Steroid preparations are divided into five categories according to how strong they are. They are termed mild or low potency (Group 1), low to medium potency (Group 2), medium or moderate potency (Group 3), high potency (Group 4), and very high potency (Group 5). The potency of the particular preparation used in each case will depend on the child's age, the severity of the eczema, the size of the affected area and what other treatment is being given. It is based on the innate potency of the drug, the concentration of it in the cream or oil base, and the base itself, which determines how effectively it is taken up by the skin.

Topical steroids work by binding to receptors in the skin which control inflammation, and thus damping it down. The creams work by alleviating the symptoms of inflammation, redness and itching, and thus allow the damaged skin to heal. With children they also help prevent the scratching which makes the symptoms worse. While steroids can be extremely effective in treating eczema in the short term, they do have a tendency to become less effective the longer they are used.

### Side-effects of steroids

Side-effects are mainly caused by excess steroids which affect the skin and get into the bloodstream. They may damage the collagen protein, which gives the skin its elasticity, and overuse can lead to thinning of the skin. These changes are very similar to those which occur with ageing. What happens is that the production of collagen slows down and falls behind the natural loss through the shedding of skin; the skin therefore becomes thinner, more transparent and more fragile, the blood vessels running through the skin become more visible and are more liable to damage, and the skin therefore bruises more easily.

If caught early, these side-effects are easily reversible. Stopping the application of steroids soon results in an increase in collagen production and the skin returns to normal. If, however, these early changes are not noticed or steroid treatment continues regardless, they can become permanent. The dermis can become badly damaged and lose its elasticity; stretch marks or *striae* appear similar to those found on the abdomen in pregnancy; and they are permanent.

The application of steroids can also cause the skin to blanch, and when they are stopped there can be a 'rebound' effect, with small blood vessels under the skin becoming more visible, a condition which can become permanent if steroids are used for too long. For this reason steroids are used as little as possible on the face. These skin changes take weeks to develop, so steroid use should be restricted to short periods to allow the skin to recover in between.

If used in large amounts, some of the steroids will inevitably be absorbed and get into the bloodstream, where they can very occasionally lead to problems. Protein metabolism can be affected, causing muscle weakness, and so can calcium metabolism, causing retarded bone growth in children.

There is a definite risk of internal side-effects when high- or very-high-potency preparations are used on children with eczema. The risk will be greatest when large quantities are used on extensive areas of the skin over a longer period. The risk will also be greater in small children, because of the greater surface area in relation to the child's weight. It is impossible to give any definite guidelines, and this is something that the doctor will have to consider in each individual case.

Group 1 preparations rarely cause any side-effects, unless they are used for long periods on a very small baby. Group 2 preparations are also unlikely to cause side-effects except in babies. Group 3 preparations could cause unwanted side-effects if used in large quantities over a long time, especially in children under five. Group 4 or 5 preparations are almost bound to cause side-effects, so they are seldom used for periods of more than a few days when the eczema is particularly severe.

Children react very individually to steroids, with some showing more side-effects at lower doses than others. Because of this, most dermatologists will therefore monitor your child's growth to make sure that it is not being retarded by the steroids.

### Administering steroids

The way that steroids are delivered to the skin, whether in a cream base or an ointment, can affect how well it is taken up. Ointment is usually used for dry skin and cream for a weepy skin. Steroid creams will almost always be prescribed by a doctor, and it is best to seek expert advice on which preparation is likely to be the best for your child. It is very important that you use the right amount, and a doctor will be able to tell you the correct dose. Hospitals use a 'finger-tip dosing unit' method for assessing the amount of steroid cream you should apply. One unit is the amount of cream from a standard tube it takes to cover an adult finger from the tip to the crease of the first joint. The dose depends on the age of the child. Getting the dose right is an important component of the treatment.

Usually steroids are used to treat a particularly bad attack and then withdrawn as the skin improves. Again, you need a doctor's advice, as stopping steroids too quickly can cause the eczema to come back worse than ever. Because of this, more powerful steroids are often used at first for a few days, then replaced with less powerful ones, each for a few days, to help avoid a relapse.

One feature of topically applied steroids is that they tend to start losing their effect after a period of regular use. How quickly this happens depends on how often the preparation is used; the more often the cream or ointment is applied, the more quickly its effectiveness will fade. The effect also seems to be more pronounced with more potent preparations, especially those in Groups 4 and 5. This is another reason why overuse of steroids is not helpful.

If the eczema is bad, the steroid cream can be used under a dressing to increase its effectiveness. This is known as occlusion and works mainly because the skin is kept moister. Polythene film can be put on the skin on top of the preparation to increase its uptake. Bandages can be put on top of this overnight to keep the cream in contact with the skin and to prevent scratching.

One of the most effective ways of using steroids is under wet dressings known as wet wraps. This technique has been used very successfully on children with severe eczema at Great Ormond Street Hospital in London. Although wet wraps can be useful with moisturizing creams and ointments, if the eczema is severe they work better when a steroid is used as well. The favoured preparation for this treatment is a diluted form of beclomethasone diproprionate. The child is bathed, cream is applied generously and the wet bandages are put on top. Some children may be frightened or resist, so it can help to get your child to help bandage a favourite doll or teddy bear first, and explain what will happen.

Very rarely oral steroids may be prescribed, but steroids given by mouth tend to cause the adrenal glands to stop their own production of cortisol. This means that if the body needs more cortisol to respond to an infection or trauma of some sort, it will be unable to produce it. Oral steroids also have a greater effect in slowing down bone growth and fluid retention, and increasing appetite and weight. Steroids can also increase blood pressure. Oral treatment is therefore only used in very severe cases, when the child's normal life is being severely affected. Some doctors will not prescribe oral steroids under any circumstances, but others will if they consider the child's quality of life is so severely affected that it is worth running the risks of adverse side-effects.

Because of the effect on growth, they are not usually advised when the child is going through puberty and the period of most rapid growth.

Prednisolone is the drug most often given orally for severe eczema. Relatively high doses are needed; most doctors give high doses initially and then move to lower and lower doses as the eczema comes under control as starting with an initial low dose may not be enough to cause an improvement.

Beclomethasone dipropionate, which was originally developed as an inhaled drug for asthma and is used in wet wraps, has also been found to be useful when given by mouth. It is quickly inactivated when it passes through the liver, so stays in the bloodstream for a shorter period than other steroids.

**Steroid preparations**
Some of the steroid preparations available are:

- **very high potency**: clobetasol propionate 0.05%, fluocinalone acetonide 0.2%, halcinonide 0.1%
- **high potency**: betamethasone valerate 0.1%, betamethasone dipropionate 0.05%, diflucortalone valerate 0.1% fluocinolone acetonide 0.025%, hydrocortisone 17-butyrate 0.1%, triamcinolone acetonide 0.1%, budeosonide 0.025%, desoxymethasone 0.25%, fluocinonide 0.05%
- **medium potency**: betamethasone valerate 0.025%, deoxymethasone 0.5%, fluocinolone acetonide 0.00625%
- **low–medium potency**: clobetasone butyrate 0.5%, flurandrenolone 0.0125%
- **low potency**: hydrocortisone or hydrocortisone acetate 0.5%, 1%, or 2.5%.

There are two new topical preparations with new steroids which are thought to bind more effectively to the steroid receptors in the skin, thus lessening that amount which is absorbed into the blood, and cutting down the risk of side-effects. One is fluticasone propionate, which is available as both a cream and an ointment. Studies with this on skin-thinning side-effects showed that there was no thinning after eight weeks of daily usage. The other is mometasone fuorate, available as a cream, an ointment and an alcohol-based scalp application. This binds tightly to the receptors in the skin and has been shown still to be present in large quantities eight hours after a single application. It can therefore be effective when applied only once a day. Studies on skin-thinning over a six-week period showed that this product produced the same amount of thinning as 1 per cent hydrocortisone, the weakest available topical steroid.

### Case Study
Amy developed quite severe eczema when she was a baby. For a long time we [her parents] resisted steroid treatments and tried other remedies, without much effect. Finally I went to the doctor for something else and was severely told off about the state of her skin, and we were referred to the hospital. She was put on strong steroids together with the emollients. At 18 months she was no better, her legs were raw and bleeding and the itching and constant scratching were terrible. We tried Ichthopaste bandages – this was a complicated business, wrapping her up, putting on steroids as well – but Amy liked the bandages, I think because it gave her some immediate relief and we were doing something for her.

## ▓ COAL-TAR AND PASTE PREPARATIONS

Grey or black creams, pastes and ointments containing tar have been used by dermatologists for over a hundred years, so their safety and effectiveness have been long established. They are still one of the most effective forms of treatment, especially in chronic eczema, when the skin has become coarse and thickened.

Preparations containing coal tar soothe the skin, reduce itching and inflammation and may help patches of eczema which are rough and thick from excessive scratching. However, they are messy, smelly, greasy, and tend to stain clothing, so are best used at night under bandages, with old nightclothes and sheets. Pre-impregnated bandages are available which are easier to use and less messy.

Tar preparations are best used under a dressing which is bandaged in place. This has the additional effect with children of preventing them from scratching and rubbing the skin. There will usually be some greyish black staining on clothing, so if the bandages are kept on during the day an old vest or other old clothing worn underneath the top layer can help.

Sticky, tar-impregnated bandages can be left on the skin for several days at a time. This is inconvenient, as the child cannot be bathed or showered and cannot swim, and may be self-conscious about the bandages, but the smooth, healed skin which emerges when they are removed can make it seem worthwhile.

Some very mild preparations containing tar have become available recently, some of which also include hydrocortisone.

Medicated bandages can be soaked in a paste containing zinc and coal tar, or a cream containing 1 per cent hydrocortisone or Ichthopaste, containing zinc oxide and ichthammol, which is milder than the coal tar. Ichthammol has a more acceptable appearance and smell, and some dermatologists recommend ichthammol pastes on top of a steroid ointment; this 'sandwich' can be a very effective treatment. The bandages can be very soothing, relieving irritation and itchiness and speeding up healing, but they often need to be covered with a dry bandage.

Other paste bandages contain calamine, which is sometimes used when the eczema is very inflamed and angry. Calamine lotion, zinc carbonate tinged pink with iron oxide, is also used in some cases to soothe eczema. It tends to have a drying effect, however, so is generally only used when the eczema is wet and oozing. There is a calamine-containing cream available which is not drying.

## ANTIHISTAMINES

Antihistamines are also used in the treatment of eczema. They help prevent inflammation but tend to produce skin reactions when applied to the skin, so although antihistamine creams and lotions are used for many types of skin irritation and itching, they are not normally advised for eczema because of the likelihood of producing an allergic response when used for any period of time. Antihistamines are therefore usually given as tablets. Their side-effect is that they tend to make you drowsy, but this can be a bonus both for the child and for parents who are worn out with lack of sleep. Some antihistamines are available which do not cause much drowsiness and can therefore be used during the day. In some children, antihistamines can produce the opposite effect, making them irritable and hyperactive.

The most commonly prescribed antihistamines are normally needed in quite high doses and should ideally be given an hour or so before your child goes to bed.

Antihistamines can cause the skin to become sensitive to sunlight. They are not addictive, although they tend to get less effective with regular use.

## ANTIBIOTICS

If the eczema becomes infected, antibiotics may be used. They are usually taken by mouth, as a suspension in a sweet-tasting liquid for young children.

The most common bacterium which infects the skin of eczematous children is *Staphylococcus aureus*. This is to be suspected when the eczema worsens with the development of weeping, pustules and crusts with a yellowish colour, or when it suddenly becomes much worse for no apparent reason. The antibiotic usually given for this is flucloxacillin, a drug similar to penicillin but more effective with this particular strain of bacterium. An alternative is erythromycin, and occasionally other antibiotics will be used.

If the eczema does not clear up fairly rapidly with the first antibiotic, a swab will usually be taken to grow the bacterium in a laboratory, identify it and see which antibiotic it is sensitive to.

The second most common strain of bacterium to infect eczema is *Group A streptococcus*. When eczema is infected with this bacterium there is usually less weeping and crusting and more redness, tenderness, and swelling. The usual antibiotics prescribed for it are phenoxymethylpenicillin, ampicillin and amoxycillin.

Antibiotics are always prescribed for a set period, usually three, five, seven or ten days. It is always important to finish the course, even though the infection seems to have cleared up after two or three days, as otherwise some bacteria can linger on and flare up again, and possibly be resistant to the original antibiotic. Antibiotics should be given at regular intervals, usually three or four times a day, as their effectiveness depends on keeping up the drug's levels in the blood.

Antibiotics may give your child mild diarrhoea but have few other side-effects. Occasionally your child may develop an allergic reaction to the drug, which may be in the form of a rash, or perhaps more severe symptoms. Once your child has been sensitized to an antibiotic, the reaction may be more severe next time, so always check with your doctor if you suspect an allergy.

Antibiotics are sometimes prescribed for external application to infected areas of eczema, rather than being given internally. The main advantage is that the risk of severe allergy is reduced. However, it is more difficult to treat infected eczema effectively with antibiotic creams and ointments because the harmful bacteria can lurk elsewhere on the skin, especially inside the nose, and spring back once the treatment ends. It is also more difficult to keep up a steady dose with skin applications. Sometimes a contact allergy to the antibiotic can also develop. Nevertheless, topical antibiotics are sometimes used for localized problem patches of infected eczema.

When a child has repeated infections of the skin, a course of continuous antibiotics over three months is sometimes recommended to prevent reinfections.

Antibiotics are obviously something of a last resort, as repeated courses may make your child more susceptible to antibiotic-resistant bacteria, and many alternative therapists believe antibiotics weaken the immune system. However, if your child's ezcema is very bad and causing a great deal of suffering, a course of antibiotics may be needed to help clear up the condition so that it can be got under control again. In severe infected eczema, your child could be at risk of septicaemia (blood poisoning) if the infection is not dealt with, so it is important to consult a doctor.

Antibiotics tend to kill off the normal bacteria which live in the gut; this is one of the reasons for the diarrhoea or loose stools which may occur when you are taking antibiotics. If your baby is still being breast-fed this should not be a problem, as breast milk promotes the growth of healthy bacteria. You can also help replace healthy bacteria after a course of antibiotics by getting your child to eat live yoghurts which contain lactobacilli – if he does not like them neat, you can mix them with fruit or honey. You should also avoid very sweet, sugary and starchy foods.

## OTHER DRUGS

### Antifungal creams

Eczema can also become infected with candida, or thrush, a fungus that is found everywhere in the air and on skin. If candida is suspected an antifungal cream containing nystatin or clotrimazole will be prescribed, often combined with topical steroids.

## Antiviral drugs

Eczema can occasionally be infected with the *Herpes simplex* (cold sore) virus. This condition is known as *Eczema herpeticum* and is very serious (*see* page 8). The child will normally need to be hospitalized and treated with the antiviral agent acyclovir.

## Anti-allergy drugs

Some drugs have been developed which help prevent the discharge of histamines in inflammation. One of these, sodium crymoglycate, has been effective when inhaled for asthma, but as yet creams containing it have not proved effective when dealing with eczema. The drug has also been tried out by mouth, but again without much effect on children with eczema.

## HOSPITALIZATION

In very severe cases of eczema, a short stay in hospital may be advised. Sometimes a week's intensive treatment of strong steroid creams and special baths can help. The hospital staff can show you and your child exactly how to apply the creams and ointments prescribed, and it is often easier to stick to a strict regime of diet and skin care when removed from the ordinary pressures of life at home. In addition, the hospital environment does not contain house-dust mites, pollen and other common allergens, the sheets are all boil-washed, and the floors and surfaces are all disinfected regularly. This clean environment often gives immediate relief to eczema sufferers.

Being admitted to hospital can have other advantages too. It can give stressed and anxious parents a break. Your child may also feel more relaxed and confident that something is going to be done to help, and can meet other children with skin complaints and realize that he is not alone, and that there are others with worse problems.

**Case Study**
At six Amy's eczema was so bad that they took her straight into hospital. This was an awful episode, because they accused me [her mother] of not doing the right things and implied that I was neglecting her treatment regime, which wasn't true. She was there for a week and her skin cleared up almost completely. While she was there they did prick tests for allergies and found she was allergic to horses and house-dust mites. When she came out of hospital the eczema came back, although we got some house-dust mite spray and sprayed the carpets, curtains and furnishings and washed and changed all the bedding. We also bought an ionizer and turned down the heating in her room, as they did a heat-monitoring test and found she was hot and slept badly at night.

Ultraviolet treatment (see below) is also advised in some cases. This can be given in hospital, as an out-patient or as part of an intensive treatment.

## LIGHT THERAPY

Some parents notice that their children's eczema improves when they go on holiday in sunnier climates and become tanned. Research has shown that exposure to ultraviolet light can improve eczema. The best results were obtained with longer-wave ultraviolet radiation combined with a drug called a psoralen which was given to the patient beforehand. Psoralens are drugs derived from plants which act to magnify the effect of ultraviolet exposure, so that treatment can be given over a short period of time. The drug can be given by mouth, applied to the skin or put in bathwater. The child then stands in a special cabinet which gives a dose of ultraviolet radiation.

This therapy (known as PUVA) has proved to be of great benefit to children, especially adolescents who have had eczema for many years and not responded to other treatments.

Unfortunately it requires very expensive equipment and highly trained staff, and it is not available in many places. Often patients have to travel long distances two or three times a week to a centre where the therapy is offered.

Another reason why this treatment is not always offered is because there is some concern that long-term side-effects may include an increase in the risk of skin cancer or premature ageing of the skin. Until the treatment has been in use for longer, these concerns will not be answered.

## TREATMENT FOR SPECIAL AREAS

### The scalp

Eczema is often found on the scalp, but is difficult to treat because the hair gets in the way. If the eczema is mild, a suitable shampoo containing a coal-tar solution can be used. In some cases an anti-yeast shampoo is helpful. These shampoos should be used at least every other day to be effective.

When more intensive treatment is needed, steroids can be given in a special liquid form to make them easier to apply. The steroids are too potent to be used for long on small children, however, and many such preparations contain alcohol which is drying and sometimes irritating to the skin.

Absorption of steroids is particularly rapid through the scalp because of its extensive blood supply. For small children, therefore, moisturizing the scalp with a water-dispersible cream is often best. Coconut oil is also good for moisturizing. It melts close to body temperature so is normally fairly solid when applied and melts once on the skin. It needs to be stored in a cool place.

### The hands

A child's hands are very commonly badly affected by eczema because they come into contact with so many substances.

Children are curious and always exploring, so it is hardly surprising that they come into contact with allergenic substances.

If your child has bad eczema, the hands should be kept out of water, especially when it contains detergents, and you should also avoid sandpits, as sand is irritating to the skin and can harbour infections. He should also be kept from touching pets, and activities like cooking and finger painting may need to be avoided too, although sometimes it is possible to do them while wearing protective gloves. The hands need to be washed to make sure they are clean and moist, and moisturizing creams should be applied regularly. Steroid ointment may be needed, and sometimes it is necessary to use a stronger steroid preparation than that used on the rest of the body. It is best to apply this at night under mittens to prevent steroids being transferred to the face.

## The feet

Some children develop eczema on the feet. The skin can be covered in blisters and peel away, and it can even become so painful that it is difficult for them to walk. Sometimes this is because the feet perspire, especially when the child is running around all day in shoes with modern synthetic linings. Some children are also allergic to the chromate used to preserve leather.

### Case Study
Fungal infections such as athlete's foot can look very like eczema, and are sometimes mistakenly treated as such. Joshua's mother recalls: 'I treated Joshua for athlete's foot, but the fungal creams didn't work. I went on and on treating him, not letting him wear trainers, and making him wear a special sock for swimming. Finally the penny dropped that it wasn't athlete's foot any more, but eczema. When we treated that the problem went away.'

## The genital area

If your child has eczema in the genital area, the itching can be a cause of embarrassment. You may also be worried that he will do some damage by too much scratching. Parents also often worry that using steroids in this area will lead to harmful effects. In fact, this is not the case and steroid creams can be applied here as everywhere else.

You should, of course, never punish or humiliate your child for scratching in this region, but simply use distraction techniques to help him to stop.

# Chapter Six

# Alternative therapies

If conventional medicine is not effective, or if you want to avoid the possible long-term side-effects of steroids and other conventional treatments, alternative therapies have much to offer. Increasingly, doctors are realizing that natural therapies can sometimes offer help where they cannot and will often support or even suggest alternative treatments.

It is sometimes difficult to prove the benefits of many alternative therapies because the role of the mind is so important in dealing with illness. It has been shown that placebos – tablets or injections which the patient believes to contain a drug but which do not – can be highly effective in relieving even severe pain, because the patient believes it will work and relaxes. Medical progress has been based on the idea of the double-blind trial in which neither the doctor nor the patients know whether they are receiving the active drug or a placebo, because if the patients think they are receiving a drug they are more likely to respond, and if the doctor believes he or she is prescribing a cure the patients somehow sense this and respond better too.

Human contact and sympathy are also very powerful in relieving symptoms and pain. This is particularly true with young children. Most parents will instinctively 'kiss it better' when their child has a cut or bruise, and a kiss, cuddle or soothing rub will often genuinely make the pain better. The simple process of applying a cream or plaster makes a big difference to the child's ability to tolerate pain and discomfort.

When you go to see a practitioner, especially an acupuncturist or homoeopath, he or she will therefore spend a great deal of time talking to you and your child, listening, and looking at her as a complete person rather than only concentrating on the symptoms. A trained homoeopath, for example, usually spends an hour and a half on the first consultation.

### Case Study

I [Sam's mother] went to see my doctor about Sam's eczema and I got five minutes with him. He looked at his skin, said, 'Yes, it's eczema, we'll prescribe this steroid cream, come back and see me if it doesn't get better.' When I went to see the homoeopath we spent an hour and a half talking about Sam's diet, his general health, our relationship, any problems in the family, everything. She was wonderfully sympathetic and seemed to understand for the first time what I was going through. She made a lot of suggestions which really helped. I came out of there for the first time feeling I was really getting somewhere.

Many of the natural therapies aim to restore the body's own balance and therefore encourage its own natural healing process. Acupuncture, aromatherapy, homoeopathy, hypnotherapy, naturopathy and reflexology, for example, have all been used on people with eczema with success in this way. It is essential that anyone seeking alternative treatments for their child should approach a qualified and experienced practitioner.

## ■ ACUPUNCTURE

The term 'acupuncture' means 'needle piercing' and is part of an ancient system of Chinese medicine. It is based on the idea that qi (pronounced 'chee'), the vital energy of the body, flows through certain channels, or meridians, creating a network throughout the whole body and linking all its parts. There are 12 main qi channels, each connected to an internal organ and named after it. When a person is healthy the qi flows smoothly through the channels, but if for some reason the flow is blocked or becomes very weak, illness occurs. The acupuncturist aims to correct the flow of qi by inserting thin needles into particular points on the channels. The treatment lasts about 20 minutes and should not cause pain, only a tingling sensation. Because most children are afraid of needles, massage, tapping or pressure with a rounded probe are often used instead. Moxibustion, the burning of herbs to stimulate the body's energy, is often also used with acupuncture.

Acupuncture can be used as preventive medicine by correcting the energy before a serious illness can occur, and also to reverse illnesses by restoring the qi.

Like many alternative therapies, acupuncture is holistic, that is, it looks at the whole person rather than simply isolating symptoms and treating them. The acupuncturist needs a detailed understanding of the patient's lifestyle, medical history, personality, work and so on before making a diagnosis. The pulse and tongue are examined to assess the body's energy and degree of illness.

Not everyone responds to acupuncture, just as not everyone can be cured by conventional medicine. But, as many will testify, it can be highly effective. Extensive research in China has shown that acupuncture is highly effective, and in China traditional and modern medicine are used equally. In Western countries, this solid research has convinced many that acupuncture does work, and it is sometimes used for anaesthesia and pain relief in Western hospitals.

### Case Study
Amy had suffered from really bad eczema since she was a baby – we [her parents] tried steroid creams, wet wraps, she even had a week in hospital. When she was seven in desperation we tried an acupuncturist. It's difficult to find one who will treat a young child but Amy was incredibly brave about the needles and everything. This was really the breakthrough and she did then start getting better. It might partially be that there was

someone there to talk to her and me – it was very different from seeing the doctor, who would say, 'Here's another tube of steroid cream and there you go.' We also went to a Chinese herbalist and she took herbs.

At nine she was much better and now she's ten she's almost completely clear, though she does sometimes get patches on her hands or behind her ears. We keep up the acupuncture and the Chinese herbalist has prescribed a cream. I think the great thing about the acupuncture and Chinese herbs was that they didn't restrict our lifestyle in the same way as the wraps and diet and everything did.

Similar to acupuncture is acupressure, where the hands, or sometimes elbows or feet, are used instead of needles.

> **Shiatsu**
> Shiatsu is a Japanese form of acupressure, in which pressure is applied to the energy lines, known as meridians. Although thumb and finger pressure is mainly used, the practitioner can also use elbows and even knees and feet.
>
> The massage stimulates the circulation, and also the body's vital energy flow. Shiatsu strengthens the nervous system and helps release toxins and deep-seated tension. On a more subtle level, it enables patients to relax deeply and get in touch with their body's own healing abilities. The patient normally lies on a futon, and it is advisable not to eat or drink much before a treatment. A feeling of calmness and well-being usually follows a treatment, and many people feel invigorated yet relaxed.

## ■ AROMATHERAPY

Aromatherapy has been described as the art and science of using essential plant oils as treatments. It is a holistic therapy, taking the mind, body and spirit into account. Oils from plants have been used medicinally for thousands of years, and of course extracts of plant oils are used in modern medicines.

Essential oils are absorbed very rapidly through the skin, and they are used in massage, in baths and in skin preparations or compresses. The essences can be diluted in a carrier oil such as pure olive oil, or in beeswax or other cream bases. A certain amount of the essential oil is also inhaled, and the scent has an effect on the mind and thus on the body. Part of the oil is also absorbed directly and rapidly into the bloodstream via the lungs. The effect of the oils, combined with soothing massage, a gentle soak in a bath and contact with the therapist is extremely beneficial. And children have a much more sensitive sense of smell than adults. They also seem to respond very quickly to essential oils.

Bathing with essential oils can be a wonderful experience and can relieve skin problems. The appropriate essential oils should be added (usually one to three drops for a child) to warm water. As essential oils do not mix well with water, the water needs to be stirred vigorously to disperse them. The child should remain in the water for ten minutes before being washed in the usual manner. Another good way to disperse oils in the bath, especially for a child with eczema, is with honey. One dessertspoonful of runny honey is an excellent disperser. Again, you need to agitate the water well.

Massage with essential oils is very useful for relaxing a child and for encouraging sleep. Children do not normally have any inhibitions about being touched, as some adults do, so they are very open and receptive to massage.

The essential oils which are recommended for eczema are bergamot, cedarwood, Roman chamomile, frankincense, geranium, lavender, rose otto, sandalwood, and sweet thyme, and the recommended carriers are avocado, calendula, carrot, sweet almond, rose hip, and white lotion.

### Case Study

Kelly had eczema behind her ears, elbows, knees and wrists, and was unable to stop scratching. She loved swimming, but the chlorine inevitably made her eczema much worse, so her mother stopped her swimming lessons. Although she had eliminated cow's milk and cheese from her diet the eczema was still bad.

The aromatherapist suggested that Kelly eat more green vegetables and fresh fruit. She mixed up 50 ml of calendula and sunflower oils with essential oils of bergamot, geranium and lavender, to be applied to the affected areas twice daily, and before swimming. After two weeks Kelly's eczema had stopped weeping and begun to heal. She was able to take up swimming again.

## ■ BIOCHEMICAL TISSUE SALTS

Biochemics is a medical system founded by a German doctor called Schuessler in the 19th century. He claimed that inner harmony could be achieved through homeostasis – a balance of the body's fluid and acid–alkali levels. This balance is easily disturbed by discrepancies in mineral and trace-element levels, and you can take small quantities of these salts to redress the balance. They are safe and easy to take and do not interact with conventional drugs.

## ■ FLOWER REMEDIES

Flowers have been used for their healing properties for thousands of years by many different cultures, including the Australian Aborigines, the ancient Egyptians, the Minoans of Crete and Native Americans. In the 1930s healing with flowers was rediscovered by Dr Edward Bach, who believed that people's emotional and psychological problems were at the root of much of their illness, and became critical of medical treatments which dealt only with the symptoms rather than the whole person. Influenced by homoeopathy, he developed 38 plant remedies from wild flowers. In the mid-1970s, Richard Katz established the Flower Essence Society in California. Many others have also been inspired to research the healing properties of their local flora.

Dr Bach made his essences by floating freshly picked flowers in a glass bowl of pure spring water in sunlight for three hours. He believed that the flower essence or energy transferred itself to the water, which he then stabilized by mixing it with an equal volume of brandy. Other flower essences are made without cutting the flowers; in Germany, for instance, Andreas Korte uses a cleaned half of a quartz geode filled with spring water which is placed in the field of the growing flower in the sun for a certain length of time to capture its energy.

The individual flower remedies chosen vary from person to person according to their personality and the exact symptoms. Bach's Rescue Remedy cream applied to eczematous skin can help calm the itching. Other remedies used are crab apple, clematis and mimulus for hypersensitive skin, and impatiens.

## ▪ HERBAL MEDICINE

Herbalism is the oldest form of medicine known. It is still used by a majority of the world's population, and in fact many modern, powerful drugs are derived from plants, such as the heart drug digitalis, which comes from foxgloves, atropine from nightshade, aspirin, which is found in willow bark, morphine from poppies and quinine from the cinchona tree.

While traditional medicine relies on extracting and purifying one active ingredient, in herbal medicine the whole plant is used, with a mixture of different ingredients. It is believed that this prevents side-effects. Herbal remedies can be chewed, swallowed, applied to the skin, put in bathwater, or inhaled. Modern herbalists often prescribe herbs in concentrated liquid form, but some use elixirs, cordials, teas, pills, ointments, bath additives and poultices. You can also grow and prepare your own herbs, but since some plants can be poisonous, you should always seek advice from a qualified herbalist, especially before giving them to young children.

Herbal remedies may vary from country to country, especially since the herbs available will differ from region to region. In the UK, traditionally herbs like burdock root, figwort, fumitory, mountain grape, nettle, pansy and red clover have a good reputation in the treatment of eczema as internal remedies. A useful tea can be made from equal parts of figwort, nettles and red clover. It should be drunk three times daily and is especially good for infantile eczema.

External remedies can also be used to reduce irritations and discomfort, but these will not heal without internal treatment too. Herbs like burdock, chickweed, comfrey, golden seal, marigold, pansy and witch hazel can be used for compresses or ointments. A marigold compress can be made by pouring a pint of boiling water on two tablespoons of dried flowers and letting it stand until cool, then soaking a compress in it and applying it to affected areas twice a day (for one hour, if your child can stand it!) Burdock makes a simple ointment; express the sap of a fresh root and mix it with petroleum jelly. It may be used on the irritated areas several times a day.

Most herbalists warn that the symptoms may get worse at first, followed by a marked improvement. This is normal with herbal remedies and should not cause anxiety.

### Russian folk remedies

A long-established herbal tradition comes from Russia. Herbal medicine was the only form of treatment available in most of pre-revolutionary Russia, where large areas were completely without any medical care. After the revolution, with the pharmaceutical industry nationalized and many drugs in short supply, and with private medical practice illegal, Russian folk medicine remained popular.

According to Paul Kourennoff, author of *Russian Folk Medicine*, Russian folk practitioners used a variety of remedies for eczema. First, the affected areas had to be kept away from sun and light by wearing a bandage or protective coat of ointment. In cases of moist eczema it was advised that all water should be avoided and the affected areas should be cleaned and bathed with decoctions of oak or pine bark only. Home-made ointments were highly recommended, including egg yolk oil, garlic-honey ointment and pipe-tar ointment.

Egg yolk oil was made by piercing the yolks of hard-boiled eggs with a slender wire or placing them in a tea-strainer and holding them over a candle. Small drops would appear which must be carefully collected and used as an ointment.

Garlic-honey ointment was made from mashed soft boiled garlic, which was combined with an equal amount of clear honey. It was applied over the affected area at night, covered with wax paper and lightly bandaged, and removed in the morning with green soap or petrol and bandaged. The following night the treatment was repeated and there were excellent results after a few days. Tar removed from a smoking pipe was often also used as ointment.

Another remedy was geranium leaf treatment. Geranium leaves were boiled in water for one hour, and the affected area was bathed in this lukewarm water, or a cloth was moistened with it and held over the affected area.

Internal remedies were also used. Throughout the Caucasus, fresh lemon juice was considered an excellent cure for all skin conditions. The juice of five lemons were taken the first day, then the amount was increased by five lemons a day until the juice of 25 lemons was given, then it was reduced to five again.

A decoction of yarrow and elder flowers in equal proportions was boiled for 20 minutes (a tablespoon of the mixture to a glass of water) and one cup taken daily.

### Chinese herbal medicine

Chinese herbal medicine is part of a sophisticated system used since ancient times. Herbs, minerals and some animal products are used to treat a wide range of diseases. The treatment is thought to restore harmony to the functions of the body, which normally means that several treatment components are given simultaneously. Unlike Western herbalists, who have a limited number of herbs at their disposal, Oriental medicine draws on a range of 4,000 herbs made up in various complex formulas. A limited number of these components are available in pill, tablet or liquid form, but most are prescribed as dried materials which are mixed to match the needs of the individual patient. Because every patient is different, the herbal mix will differ from one to another. Usually the treatment is prepared by boiling the herbs and other dried materials with water for a specified period, straining off the liquid, cooling, and then giving it to the patient.

The practitioner of Chinese herbal medicine will be looking for a pattern of disharmony, a blockage or disturbance of the patient's energy. These patterns are recognized by a combination of symptoms, mental states, non-verbal behaviour, physiological signs and a reading of both tongue and pulse.

Several years ago several dermatologists and the National Eczema Society heard that some people were being very successfully treated with Chinese herbal medicine in London. Trials into the effectiveness of the treatment were carried out with adults at the Royal Free Hospital and with children at the Great Ormond Street Hospital for Children.

The children who took part in the study were carefully selected; they had widespread eczema which had not responded to conventional treatment but was not obviously infected or weepy. The taste of the remedies was a problem, and in fact children under four could not be persuaded to take it voluntarily. The study did show however that the Chinese herbal treatment was much more effective than the placebo, showing a substantial improvement in about 70 per cent of patients, with only 30 per cent showing no worthwhile benefit. Most of the improvement was apparent by the fourth week of treatment. The study also discovered that the herbs used did not contain any steroids, so this was not responsible for the benefit seen.

Research is now going on to identify the active components of the herbs used so as to devise a more palatable form of treatment. While no toxic effects were found from the treatment, the anxiety remains that a small number of people might develop side-effects with long-term treatment, and this anxiety was heightened by reports of occasional cases of hepatitis in patients taking Chinese herbal treatment for atopic eczema, which may or may not be coincidental.

### Evening primrose oil

Evening primrose oil has been found by some to be helpful in treating eczema. It is a natural oil derived from the seeds of specific varieties of the evening primrose plant, which is rich in the essential fatty acid gamma-linoleic acid (GLA).

GLA is normally made by the body from the fatty acid linoleic acid which occurs widely in a normal diet. It is needed by the body to maintain a healthy skin and lack of it can make the skin dry and scaly. It has been found that people with atopic ezcema are less able to convert the linoleic acid in their diet into GLA, and this could be a reason for their skin problems. It makes sense therefore to take GLA directly. GLA is not suitable for babies under one year old, however.

Studies into the effectiveness of evening primrose oil have not been conclusive, with some trials showing a marked improvement in those treated with GLA and others showing none. There is however a lot of anecdotal evidence that GLA can be beneficial for children and adults with eczema. It is best to buy a brand of evening primrose oil tablets or capsules which has been tested for purity and where it is easy to measure the dose.

## HOMOEOPATHY

Homoeopathy is the best-known of the alternative therapies, and it is growing in popularity. A distrust of powerful drugs which have side-effects and may harm the body and a desire to be treated as a whole person and not just a body with specific symptoms are two reasons why people are increasingly turning to it.

Homoeopathy is a system of treatment using medicine according to the principle of 'like cures like'. It was developed as a science by a German physician, Samuel Hahnemann, who noticed that quinine, which produces the same symptoms as malaria, could be used to cure it. The symptoms of a disease often show how the body is attempting to heal itself – catarrh is used to clear foreign organisms from the respiratory tract, vaginal discharges from the reproductive tract, and so on. Homoeopathy is based on this observation that substances which cause certain symptoms can also be used to cure them. However, used in conventional doses many of these substances can be toxic, so in homoeopathy they are increasingly diluted to render them safe. The medicines are diluted by stages in an alcohol and water solution, and vigorously shaken mechanically in between, in a process known as 'potentization'.

The potency of a homoeopathic remedy refers to the extent and number of times the original extract has been diluted during the preparation. For example, Arnica 6c has been prepared by adding one drop of the original alcoholic extract to 99 drops of a solution of water and alcohol and shaken vigorously. One drop of this is added to another 99 drops, and so on, six times. The higher the degree of dilution, the greater the potency.

Critics of homoeopathy hold that some preparations have been so diluted that not even one molecule of the original substance can be contained in the solution, and therefore it is impossible that it could have any effect. Homoeopaths believe that during potentization the properties of the substance being diluted is somehow imprinted on the molecules of the solution carrying it. There is no conventional scientific explanation of how this could happen, but then there are other things which modern science cannot explain.

Some scientific studies have been carried out to try to 'prove' whether homoeopathy is effective or not, but since the mind is so powerful in influencing illness this is very difficult. Many people, however, believe from experience and observation that it does work, and it certainly cannot have any harmful consequences, so it is certainly worth trying even if you are sceptical.

One study showed that 90 per cent of children with atopic eczema were significantly improved after homoeopathic treatment. However, it was carried out over two and a half years, so it could be argued that the symptoms were likely to improve in any case. There was no comparison in this study with children who had not received treatment.

Because homoeopathy is holistic, the patient's medical history, lifestyle, temperament and feelings will be taken into account. Because of this, there is no one remedy which will be useful for everyone; the remedy has to be matched to the person. In addition, the particular form the symptoms take will also affect what is prescribed. Because everyone is different, and particularly because eczema can develop into a serious condition, you should always consult a professional homoeopath if your child's symptoms are severe, or else seek conventional medical treatment.

Eczema is viewed by homoeopaths as a deep-seated disorder, and it is always recommended that you see a practitioner rather than treating it yourself using remedies purchased from health shops or pharmacies. Homoeopaths also believe that suppressing the eczema with steroids or other remedies can lead to asthma or other allergic conditions developing later on.

Patients using homoeopathy are often warned that their symptoms may get worse before they get better, and a 'healing crisis' is often observed. If symptoms become really severe, however, further advice should be sought.

**Common homoeopathic remedies for eczema**
While every child and every case is different, and two people with the same condition will not necessarily get the same treatment, there are some common remedies used:

- **Graphites** if there is cracked and oozing skin which burns and itches
- **Petroleum** if the itch is worse at night

- **Dulcamara** for weeping and crusted eczema which is made worse by damp
- **Arsenicum Album** for dry, itchy skin made worse by cold
- **Sulphur** for intense itching made worse by heat
- **Natrum Muriaticum** for eczema with greasy skin and raw patches, especially around the hairline
- **Calcarea carbonicum** for eczema symptoms associated with constipation

### Case Study

Lucy had suffered from severe eczema since she was five months old. She had tried the standard treatments, moisturizers, steroid creams and tar wraps. By the time she was six, her mother in desperation turned to a homoeopath.

For the first time she felt that she was getting somewhere. The homoeopath talked to her for an hour and a half at the first appointment, talking about Lucy, her health, her lifestyle and the stresses the family were under. Until then Lucy had had only short, ten-minute sessions with her doctor and dermatologists. A short while after the homoeopathic treatment began, the eczema started to improve. Lucy's mother feels that the combination of the homoeopathic remedies and the changes to their lifestyle that they adopted was responsible for this. Lucy no longer suffers from eczema.


## HYPNOTHERAPY

Hypnosis immediately conjures up and image of a man in a black suit waving a watch before your eyes and then making you do things you would not normally do. Nothing could be further from the truth as far as hypnotherapy is concerned. Hypnosis is in fact a natural state which we all experience, and is normally called dozing or daydreaming. It is not being asleep or unconscious; it is in fact self-induced and anyone who wants to can let it happen. It is experienced normally as a very relaxed, floating or pleasant feeling and can also make one feel energized and alert.

Hypnotherapy means using hypnosis to work directly with the subconscious mind, channelling its resources to achieve a positive change. The subconscious mind controls our feelings and behaviour, and often a negative cycle is set up which limits us. As soon as the eczema starts to flare up and the skin itches unbearably, for example, the sufferer may immediately feel all the emotions of despair, depression, anger, resentment and so on, and these negative emotions may be worse that the illness itself. Tension, stress and worry all make it harder for us to heal ourselves.

Hypnotherapy has been used very successfully to deal with pain and chronic illness, and it can certainly be used to help overcome some of the negative aspects of eczema, and in particular to stop your child scratching and thus making the condition worse. The hypnotherapist can teach your child ways of distracting her attention from the itchiness of her skin. The therapy can work well with children, usually over the age of seven, as their powerful imagination can be harnessed. When the skin starts itching, especially when trying to go to sleep, your child can imagine a cool, snowy landscape or some other pleasant environment where the skin will not itch. Or she can be taught to imagine the itch moving to a particular place on the body, like one finger, and rubbing this will relieve the itch.

The therapist can also try post-hypnotic suggestion, the technique which is most familiar from stage hypnotists. First he or she gets the child into a deeply relaxed, trance-like state, when an idea or instruction can be planted into the mind – something like: 'When your skin starts itching at school, sit very still, and then press one finger on the part that itches most; this will make the itch go away.'

## ▨ PSYCHOTHERAPY AND COUNSELLING

It is not always possible to differentiate between a counsellor and a psychotherapist – some practitioners could be described as either. There are also psychoanalysts, and many different schools of psychoanalysis – the Freudian and Jungian are the best known, but there are also Kleinian, Adlerian, Rogerian, and so on. One also comes across psychiatrists (medical doctors who then specialize in psychiatry), psychologists (who are not medically trained, but have a degree in psychology and may specialize in educational, clinical or academic psychology) and behaviourists. But all counsellors, psychotherapists and analysts should have had an intensive training and appropriate qualifications.

Psychotherapy is not normally advisable for young children. This is because a young child cannot really consent to the treatment, and may not understand the full implications of what is going on, and psychotherapy is normally only helpful when the client has consented to it and wants to take part. Children who have psychotherapy forced on them may resent it bitterly and it may actually be damaging to them.

This is not to say that in some cases counselling or talking to a child with eczema may not be helpful. Often it can help not only to relieve the distress of the condition but also to look at ways of managing your child's stress, emotions and lifestyle. The whole family may also benefit from some kind of counselling or therapy when the eczema is causing severe problems within the family or straining the relationship between parents and child. Sometimes parents may need counselling from marriage guidance agencies if the strain of coping with their ill child is causing problems in their relationship.

There are also many treatments available to help adults who are suffering from stress (see pages 31–2).

## REFLEXOLOGY

Reflexology is a system of foot massage which has been practised in most ancient cultures from China to North America. A gentle but firm finger pressure and a special massage technique are applied to areas of the feet and lower legs which correspond to the glands, organs and other parts of the body. The blocking of energy paths results in imbalance and disease, as explained under 'Acupuncture' on page 58, and tensions in the body manifest themselves in the feet. By applying gentle pressure with the hands to relevant areas of the foot, toxins can be removed from the body and circulation improved, restoring the free flow of energy and nutrients to the body cells.

Reflexology is not a diagnostic therapy, but it can indicate if certain organs or glands are under pressure. It can often detect injuries which occurred years ago, and also can detect weaknesses which have not yet developed into disease.

Treatment sessions usually take between 50 and 80 minutes, and the number of treatments required varies according to the individual and the nature of the disorder. During treatment the patient may feel a slight discomfort on certain parts of the foot, and he or she may feel tired and lethargic at first, but this followed by a renewed sense of wellbeing. Reflexology can create a deep sense of relaxation, which can encourage the body's own healing processes.

## REIKI

This is an ancient Japanese therapy in which hands are laid on the body to promote relaxation and natural healing. The patient simply relaxes and enjoys the warmth of the practitioner's hands over the area of pain or need. Reiki can help a large number of ailments, including a variety of skin complaints.

## SPA TREATMENT

In Victorian times spas used to be one of the main treatments for many skin diseases, and in some countries they are still frequently used today. The Victorians developed many spa towns and people would go to drink the waters or bathe in them. Spa treatments can still be very effective.

Spa waters contain many dissolved minerals which can help with eczema. In one highland spring in Scotland, for example, the waters were found to contain 19 cubic inches of sulphurated hydrogen per gallon, and a well in Edinburgh is coated with a black oily material which is coal tar – still used for the treatment of eczema today.

Amy's mother recalls how bathing in spa water helped her daugher:

### Case Study

One thing that did work to help Amy's ezcema was when we went on holiday to a spa in Italy. There were hot springs and it was a famous place for skin disorders. Amy could bathe there and it worked immediately. We went to the baths for two weeks and she bathed every day and her skin improved dramatically. I remember Amy saying, 'If we lived in Italy I wouldn't have eczema.'


## ▦ VISUALIZATION

This is a technique which can help people with recurring illness or who suffer from continual pain. It is a way of focusing the mind in such as way as to help the sufferer relax and think positive thoughts which can help ease pain or make it seem less hard to bear.

The techniques of relaxation may be familiar to many mothers who have attended antenatal classes, which often include relaxation exercises. The technique is to tense and then relax all the parts of the body, concentrating first on the feet, and progressing up the body to end with the head. It is possible to teach these techniques to children and especially to teenagers, to help them sleep and cope with stress.

With younger children, you can use their imagination to help them relax before using visualization. If your child is frantic with the desire to scratch, go through a visualization technique. Tell her to shut her eyes, and then to imagine the skin turning from an inflamed red to a cool, smooth blue. She could imagine being in a cool place, perhaps playing with snow, swimming in cold water or cuddling an icy snowman. There is some evidence that under hypnosis parts of the body can become cooler or warmer if this is suggested to the person in a trance, so there may be some direct effect.

# Chapter Seven

# As they grow

The problems caused by eczema often vary according to the child's stage of development, and so, therefore, will the strategies for dealing with them.

## ◼ BABIES

Eczema normally appears in the first year of life, after the first few weeks or so. Some parents notice that their baby seems to have a dry and sensitive skin, which easily forms a rash, perhaps nappy rash. In other cases the rash appears later, perhaps when the baby has been weaned onto solid foods or onto cow's milk.

The first signs of eczema may be a slight redness on the skin, especially the cheeks, and the baby may be irritable, try to rub or scratch, and sleep badly. In fact, one of the main problems for parents of babies with eczema is getting enough sleep. The baby will frequently wake often in the night, disturbed by the itching. Moreover, if they cry for too long, they will inevitably become hot and sweaty, which makes the eczema worse, so the parents rush in at the first sound of crying, and walk them up and down to send them back to sleep again after feeding. Nappies will need to be changed frequently if the skin underneath is sore, and so will clothes. Sometimes a bath is needed in the middle of the night, followed by applications of creams to calm the skin down and allow the baby to sleep. All this can mean many broken nights.

Solving the sleep problem is probably the most important factor for people whose babies have eczema. They can cope with almost anything during the day if they get a good night's sleep, and the babies can be distracted from their sore and itching skin by activity, going for walks, being carried, being fed, being soothed and rocked. But at night there are no distractions, and you may be dying to sleep, exhausted and at the end of your tether.

Some parents solve the problem by taking their babies into bed with them. There is no reason at all why you should not do this – many parents do it even with healthy babies, and if your child needs extra attention it may be easier to provide this when he is sleeping next to you. Sometimes the parents take it in turns to sleep with the child so that they can each get some sleep during their 'off-duty' times.

Some people, however, find it worse to sleep with their child because of the constant, albeit low-level, disturbance of the baby whimpering and scratching. There is no point in feeling guilty if you cannot do what you feel you should; every family has to work out its own solutions and do what suits it best.

A baby with eczema may develop poor sleep patterns, so the disrupted sleep familiar to most parents of small babies continues far longer. Everyone has light periods of sleep around the time of dreaming, and babies with eczema may surface just enough to realize that they are itching and start scratching, which then wakes them up. Many wake every hour or two throughout the night and need attention to get them back to sleep. Although your baby will need to know that you are there and be soothed, it can help to keep this to a minimum once the baby gets a bit older. Some grow to like this parental attention in the night and exploit the condition. Babies can usually catch up on some of the lost sleep during the day but the parents cannot. Kindness but firmness is usually the best policy.

When your baby wakes he can be fed or offered a drink, depending on age, soothed and creamed if necessary, and then returned to cot or bed. If the crying continues, you can go back at 10- or 15-minute intervals to calm and reassure your child, but do not pick him up. In that way he will learn that night-time is for sleeping. This technique, known as sleep training, usually works, but it can be hard to put into practice. Most doctors will refer you to a sleep clinic, usually based in your local hospital or at a child health clinic, if your child's sleep problem seems to be dominating your life.

There are other things you can do to help your child to sleep better. It is important that he does not become overheated at night, as this can make the itching worse. If you have your baby in bed with you it may help if you are not both huddled up under a thick duvet, but under a sheet covered with a cellular cotton blanket. It also helps to keep the room cooler than normal at night.

Scratching causes much of the skin damage in infantile eczema, so keeping the nails short is very important. It is easiest to cut them when they are soft just after a bath, or you can bite them. Scratch mittens help, but they often come off; cotton sleepsuits with built-in mittens are best.

Nappies also can be a problem. If the skin is sensitive, the baby is more likely to develop nappy rash if urine or stools are left on the skin for any length of time. Some children react to the bleaches or chemicals in some disposable nappies, and others to detergents used in washing terry nappies. It is best to experiment and find out whether disposables or terries are best for your baby. You may also need to change the nappy more often than usual. You should also use a cream such as zinc and castor oil or Vaseline on the nappy area to help protect the skin. On the other hand, the eczema may sometimes be less severe in the nappy area than elsewhere, because the moisturizing creams together with the urea in the baby's urine help to keep the skin moist.

### Case Study
Severe eczema in a baby is very distressing, especially when the face is affected as it often is. A mother recalls: 'People would look into the pram oohing and aaahing and then suddenly recoil.

People would ask me if the rash was catching and what was wrong with him. Other people would imply that I wasn't looking after him properly or his skin couldn't be so bad. At one stage I used to hate taking him out because I dreaded the comments.'

Alison, whose first baby had eczema, remembers her feelings of helplessness:

### Case Study
The worst thing is you can't explain. He was in distress and pain and there was nothing I could do to help him. Once his eczema got infected and I couldn't do anything to help – he would cry if I left him and cry if I picked him up because it hurt him to be touched. I couldn't say, never mind, it'll get better, and you'll grow out of it – which he has.

## TODDLERS

The toddler period, from 18 months to three years, is notorious as the period of tantrums. This is the stage at which young children begin to assert themselves for the first time as independent beings apart from their mothers or other carers. One of the most common words used by children of this age is 'No'. Another very common phrase is 'Me do it'. Children will want to tie their own shoelaces, climb onto things, put on their own clothes, and they will resist all interference. But sometimes, especially when they are tired or hungry, it will all be too much for them. Then they will vent their frustration with a full-blown tantrum, rejecting help, but unable to do what they want either.

Even children as young as this can realize that they can use their eczema as a weapon for getting attention and to avoid doing things they do not want to do. They may learn that scratching themselves gets an instant response from you. If children become hot and bothered their eczema often gets worse, so they learn to get hot and bothered because it gets them what they want. They may find that impossible, aggressive or dangerous behaviour is excused because their parents feel sorry for them because of the eczema.

It may be hard, but tantrums which involve scratching have to be ignored just like others. This does not mean that you should be harsh with your child. The best, quickest and kindest way to deal with tantrums is to leave the child alone, distract him at the earliest opportunity, and carry on as usual as soon as the tantrum stops. Ignoring the screams and getting on with what was going on before can also help your child learn that tantrums do not work. Screaming, shouting or hitting your child will usually make the tantrum worse. Moreover, children prefer negative attention to no attention at all, so this will often encourage them to try the same tactic again. Calmness is hard to achieve, but the best response.

Of course it is best to avoid tantrums whenever possible. You can do this by ensuring that you do not let your child become too stressed or too hungry, and by anticipating when a tantrum is about to happen and defusing it. You can do sometimes do this by compromise; if a task is proving too much, you can say, 'Let me do this bit and you do that bit', and it sometimes works.

Controlling scratching can be very difficult. It is no good just saying 'Stop scratching' when your child is distraught with the itching. You can help by saying, 'Let me rub it for you.' You can then gently rub the skin instead of letting your child scratch. Encourage him to do the same and it may become a habit. Again, distraction often helps.

One thing you can do is keep your child's fingernails very short to minimize damage. As I have said, it is easiest to do this when the nails are soft after a bath. Filing is better than cutting because it keeps the ends smooth. If your child really hates having this done and struggles, you can try doing it when he is asleep, as toddlers and young children normally sleep very deeply and may not be disturbed.

You can also put on an emollient cream as soon as your child starts scratching and say that this will make it better – which it will. If you give him a little cream to rub in, it will help him feel more independent and in control. You can also put cotton gloves or socks on the hands at night or even wrap them in bandages to stop your child scratching and causing damage while asleep.

Dietary restrictions can begin to be difficult at this age. Up to the age of 18 months your child will have accepted what you have provided without question. Now, however, he will have become aware of delicious forbidden foods such as some biscuits, sweets and cakes. If children see others being given treats they are not allowed, or if they are offered something by another adult and see their parents refusing it, they will usually become very angry and frustrated. They will not be able to understand that the food is bad for them. They will only know that their parents are denying them what they want and that this can only be because they do not love them. They will be even more frustrated, and the irritating rash can mean they have a shorter fuse than many toddlers.

### Case Study

It is important to stress to other people caring for your child how important the diet is. 'When Joshua was at the working mothers' nursery they were very good at supervising him, washing his hands when he came into contact with anything he reacted to, and watching his diet, but it was hard. He wasn't allowed cake and other treats so they used to give him something else. I [his mother] used to keep a treat tin at home with things he could eat for when other children were having treats. I discovered how to make an eggless cake and we bought eggless ice cream.'

## PRE-SCHOOL AND SCHOOL

Starting at pre-school, nursery or school can be quite a stressful time for your child and at least in the short term this can make the eczema worse. Until your child goes to pre-school or nursery school or starts school he will probably have been very much protected. He will probably have met people mainly at home or in the houses of other people who know about or have been warned about the eczema, and are unlikely to make hurtful remarks. At school, however, strange children may stare, ask why your child's skin is funny, and make other remarks that draw his attention to the condition.

Children can be notoriously cruel to anyone who is different from themselves. One girl of six with severe eczema remembers that other children in her class avoided her, and pretended that if they touched her they would catch what they called 'Pippa's fever'. This child was too upset to tell any adults what was going on.

### Case Study

In some cases, sensitive teachers can deal with the problem very effectively. Alex's eczema was very bad, especially on her face and scalp. The other children used to make remarks which upset her to such an extent that she did not want to go to school. Her mother had a word with the teacher, who got the children to sit on the mat and talked to them about how everyone has things that they are sensitive about and how to deal with things people say. She said that she used to have sticky-out ears and was teased about that. She mentioned other things which led to teasing or misunderstanding, such as being too tall or small or fat or thin, and mentioned conditions like eczema, what caused it, what to do about it, and so on, and explained that this was what Alex had. One boy talked then about his brother who had asthma and another said that he used to have eczema as a baby. As a result of this, the questions stopped and the children became sympathetic towards Alex, who became much happier in school.

It is very important that before your child starts nursery or school, you talk to the teachers about any problems and how to deal with them. This can help smooth the transition for your child, and help the teachers and other staff to be aware of activities which might exacerbate the condition. Sand play, water play and some other activities may be bad for the skin. There may be an allergy or intolerance to some foodstuffs when the children prepare food or eat what they have cooked, especially when baking, and your child also may react to some modelling materials. Some children also react to protective plastic gloves and plastic overalls, so these may not solve the problem either.

As your child grows older, some other activities will need to be restricted, so that contact with substances to which he or she is allergic is avoided. This can mean restrictions on playing with animals, on visits to the zoo, on visiting other houses, on swimming, and on eating certain foods.

### Swimming

It is best if possible to allow the child to take part in normal sports and activities. Swimming presents a particular problem, however, because the chlorine in swimming pools often aggravates the skin. In modern pools which are heated and covered over, the chlorine level is high not only in the water but in the air surrounding the pool.

If your child goes swimming, therefore, it is best to put on a layer of Vaseline or moisturizing cream to protect the skin before he goes into the water. After the swim, he should shower thoroughly and you should wash his hair so that chlorine does not stay there to irritate the scalp, back of the neck and face. You or he should also rub on cream on his skin in the shower to wash away all traces of chlorine and to moisturize the skin.

Some children react to certain kinds of chlorinating agents but not to others. If you find that your child's eczema flares up more in certain swimming pools than others, avoid those which produce a severe reaction and check on which chlorinating agent is used before you go to a new pool.

Sea-water bathing can also be a problem if your child's skin is inflamed and especially if the skin is broken, as the salt can sting unbearably. Again, protecting the skin with Vaseline or moisturizers can help.

## Sports

Taking part in vigorous sports can also be a problem for children with eczema. Inflamed skin tends to perspire less easily, making it harder for them to stay cool. Perspiration is salty and this can sting the skin, and hot, sweaty skin can make them itch unbearably. In addition, many sports clothes are made of synthetic fabric which traps perspiration close to the skin and helps prevent evaporation – this is especially true of the 100 per cent polyester football shirts so beloved of small boys, and many girls' leotards and leggings contain artificial fibres which help them to cling tightly to the skin and make the child overheat.

Sports footwear can also be a problem. Modern trainers have synthetic linings which tend to make the foot hot and sweaty and will aggravate eczema. Most children with eczema do better if they wear cotton socks and leather shoes with natural soles. Good-quality towelling sports socks made of cotton are a good idea as they will tend to absorb moisture and draw it away from the skin. Trainers and sports socks should always be changed after the sports session is over.

Showering to wash perspiration off the skin and relieve itching is always a good idea after sport. At school children may be expected to shower after games, but if not, it is a good idea to make sure it is possible for your child to do so or to wash down. If this is not possible, you may have to get your child to have a shower as soon as he comes home.

Encouraging your child and his school to start other forms of exercise may help. Yoga or tai chi, for example, will not make your child perspire and will also be very beneficial.

Some children will have to undress or change for school sports activities. This can be very embarrassing for a child whose eczema is bad, especially if it is worse in areas which are normally covered up. You can help by teaching your child ways of dressing and undressing which minimize exposure. It is also a good idea to give him the self-confidence to deal with any remarks that may be made.

It is also very important that once your child starts school you do not neglect the skin-care regime, which often has to be fitted into a busy day. It can help to start the day earlier so that you can bath your child and moisturize the skin before he goes to school. While your child is young, it may be necessary to go into school at lunchtime to apply creams or wash his hands, if the school are not able to take adequate care.

### The school environment

Schools are normally sympathetic to children who have any illness which requires special attention. However, while some teachers are happy to give the children any medicines they may be taking and to help by rubbing on creams during the school day, others require the parent to come in to administer these. It will help if you teach your child to rub on creams and take any medicine as soon as he or she is able to take this responsibility.

If your child is on a special diet, it is often a good idea to provide a packed lunch so that you can be sure he is not eating anything likely to cause a reaction. This does not have to be boring sandwiches; with a bit of imagination you can provide a wide variety of foods. Many school meals are not very nutritious or good for children, involving staples like chips, burgers and pizza. It is not hard to provide more interesting meals than this, and in some cases children with packed lunches have been the envy of others who have to eat the boring school lunches!

However, at some schools eating the communal meal is an important part of socializing and learning about table manners, and in some, children who have packed lunches have to sit at separate tables. So it is best to talk to your school and find out the best solution in your individual case.

If your child has school lunches it is important to make sure that the school knows that it is important that the necessary dietary restrictions are kept to. This may mean informing lunchtime assistants and asking them to provide alternative foods when the main menu contains a large number of items to which your child is allergic so as to avoid his diet being adversely affected.

It can also be a good idea to check that your child sits in the coolest part of the classroom, away from radiators or other sources of heat. If the eczema seems worse at school, it may be worth investigating whether there is something in the classroom which may be causing an allergic reaction.

It is important to talk to your child's teacher about the eczema – what situations will exacerbate it, and how it will be made much worse with scratching. However, endless cries of 'Stop scratching!' from the teacher or classmates will not have any effect and your child may need to leave the room for a short period to calm down and maybe rub cream onto the skin. Ask the teacher also to encourage him to pat or rub the itch rather than scratching.

Because your child is more likely to pick up infections when the skin is raw or broken, ask the teacher to make sure that he does not have contact with children who have cold sores or impetigo. There is also a very small risk if your child has broken skin and comes into contact with the blood of anyone infected with HIV, the AIDS virus. The risk *is* very small, but it is worth mentioning in case there is an HIV positive child at the school.

Some children with eczema may fall behind with schoolwork for a number of reasons. They may be distracted by the itching, or if they are taking antihistamines they may become drowsy and find it hard to concentrate on what is being taught. Some children will miss school for days at a time when the eczema is particularly bad, or if they have to go into hospital. They may also have time off school for doctor's appointments and regular check-ups with the dermatologist. If you think your child's education is suffering, then talk to the teacher or the head. Extra help may be available to help children who have fallen behind with reading or other areas of schoolwork. There may also be extra help you could provide yourself at home.

## Case Study

Another problem that can arise is that teachers' expectations of children with eczema, who have particular problems, may be lower. 'Simon's hands were very badly affected when he was first learning to write. There were times when he could hardly hold the pencil. He was absent from school from time to time and when he was there he was often tired and sleepy because of endless sleepless nights. The teachers saw this boy with cracked and weeping hands doing his best and they probably felt it was good enough. They didn't push him to form his letters correctly or hold his pencil the right way. It was difficult later to teach him to re-learn good writing skills because the undecipherable scrawl had become instinctive.'

In severe cases, there are some special schools which cater for children with eczema and asthma. Such schools provide an environment in which dust and other allergens are controlled, individual diets can be monitored and supervised, medical care is on hand and physiotherapy is provided. Fitness programmes including swimming are built into the school day. Individual programmes can help the child who has missed a lot of school to 'catch up' and special one-year courses are also offered to students who have been left behind in their schooling.

While parents might feel they have failed if they send their child away to school, there are some cases in which it is beneficial. Children can meet others with similar problems and realize that they are not alone. Especially when they are becoming teenagers and need to become more independent, spending time away from their parents can give them more confidence. Parents are able to visit and are kept regularly informed of their child's progress by the school.

## ▨ TEENAGERS

As children grows older and become teenagers, they may become more severely affected by their appearance. The average teenager will spend hours in front of the mirror despairing at the appearance of a tiny spot, so it is not hard to imagine how disabling it can be to have a rash all over the face and body. Teenage girls may have to be careful about which cosmetic products they use, as some will irritate the skin. If you have eczema on your face it is tempting to cover it up, but this can sometimes make the skin worse. It's important to help your child find suitable products such as hypo-allergenic cosmetics which will not irritate the skin. This also applies to the deodorants, perfume, and skin and hair products which boys and girls start using at puberty.

When your child is about 12 his attitude towards you will normally change considerably. This often coincides with the start of secondary school and the adoption of a much more independent attitude. Your child will now need to take on a lot of the responsibility for putting on creams, keeping to a diet and caring for the skin. It will be much more difficult to liaise with the school and meals are not normally supervised.

Your child may now resent your efforts to help: 'Stop fussing', 'Leave me alone', 'I'll do it later' and 'I know what I'm doing' become common cries. This can be very upsetting for parents who have been taking great care of their child's skin-care regime and diet, and fears – or even sees – that it is getting worse without their vigilance. However, it is important to let go and let the child take more responsibility. Perhaps they need to find out for themselves that their skin will get worse if they do not cream themselves regularly.

Further, as children starts to enter puberty and become aware of their changing bodies, they may not want their parents to look at or touch them in the same way, and this is natural and understandable. As one mother said:

I used to cream Sam in the shower and rub him all over with aqueous cream. Then when he turned 12 suddenly the bathroom door was locked. I wasn't allowed in and I wasn't allowed to see him without any clothes on. I no longer knew how much cream he was using and whether he was using it properly, and I couldn't see whether the eczema was getting worse or not.

Communicating with the school can also be a problem. Many teenagers do not want parents to make a special fuss about their eczema, and may resist their attempts to talk to teachers or write to the school about it. There can be other problems too.

Examinations usually take place at the hottest time of the year and when pollen counts are high, which is very bad news for children who suffer from atopic eczema, asthma and hay fever. Some schools may allow such pupils to take the examination in a cool, quiet room, away from a window. And if they are taking antihistamines which will affect their performance, or have infected skin and are taking antibiotics, teachers may inform the examining board, who can take this into account if their marks are on the borderline between grades or between success and failure. In severe cases, if your child is in hospital it can even be arranged for examinations to be taken there. It may also be possible to arrange for your child to sit examinations earlier or later than usual, in the winter.

## Case Study

Shelley's eczema was a problem for her well into her teens: 'I had very bad eczema as a baby and my mum tried everything, creams, steroids, bandages and so on. I even went into hospital when I was seven. It then got much better but it started up again when in my second year at secondary school. The school moved buildings and I don't know whether that had something to do with it. I became very self-conscious about it as everyone stared at my face and asked me what was the matter with it. My hands were bad too. I missed a lot of school. I took antihistamines which made me very sleepy. If I used strong steroid creams on my face it got better but then I

worried about what it was doing to my skin. I got very behind
with my schoolwork especially after I went into hospital again.

'At one stage I couldn't really go dancing or anything
because if I got sweaty and there was lots of smoke around my
skin just flared up terribly. I hated going swimming because I
was afraid that everyone could see the eczema all over my
body. Then I went to counselling about it and I also started
seeing a homoeopath. She said it was important not to let it
rule my life so now I make a lot more effort to go out and do
things with my friends, my eczema seems better, and I'm a lot
less bothered about what people will think.'

# Conclusion

If you have read this far you will now know that there are a wide variety of treatments, both conventional and alternative, to help improve your child's eczema. And time is also on your side, because in the great majority of cases eczema improves as the child grows older and it eventually goes away altogether. You may have to try several treatments to see which is best for you, but there is every chance that you will find something that works for your child and provides significant relief. Further, making changes to your child's and indeed the whole family's diet to make it healthier, and making changes in your lifestyle to remove areas of stress, can make your child and your family healthier and happier in the long run.

And although there will be problems, you may well find that in caring for your child you become closer than you might have been, and that your child also develops qualities of will-power, resilience, sensitivity and compassion which a child who has no problems to overcome might not do.

# Further reading

## ON ECZEMA

Atherton, David J., *Eczema in Childhood – the facts*, Oxford University Press, Oxford, 1995

Lewis, Jenny, *The Eczema Handbook*, Vermilion, London, 1994

Lask, Bryan, *Atopic Eczema*, British Society for Paediatric Dermatology, London, 1995

Meredith, Sheena, *The Natural Way: Eczema*, Element Books, Shaftesbury, 1994

## ON ALTERNATIVE THERAPIES

*Back to Balance: A Self-help Encyclopaedia of Eastern Holistic Remedies*, Kodansha International Limited, US and Japan, 1996/Newleaf, England, 1996

Carter, Jill and Edwards, Alison, *The Elimination Diet Cookbook*, Element Books, Shaftesbury, 1997

—, *The Rotation Diet Cookbook*, Element Books, Shaftesbury, 1997

Castro, Miranda, *Homeopathic Guide, Mother and Baby*, Pan Books, London, 1992

Harvey, Clare and Cochrane, Amanda, *The Encyclopaedia of Flower Remedies*, Thorsons, London, 1995

Kourennoff, Paul, *Russian Folk Medicine*, W H Allen, London, 1970

Lever, Dr Ruth, *Acupuncture for Everyone*, Penguin, London, 1987

Pines, Dinora, *A Woman's Unconscious Use of Her Body*, Virago Press, London, 1993

Price, Shirley and Price Parr, Penny, *Aromatherapy for Babies and Children*, Thorsons, London, 1996

# Useful addresses

## AUSTRALIA

**Australian Natural Therapists
Association**
PO Box 308
Melrose Park
South Australia 5039
Tel: 8297 9533

## CANADA

**Canadian Holistic Medical
Association**
700 Bay Street
PO Box 101, Suite 604
Toronto
Ontario M5G 1Z6
Tel: 416 599 0447

## UK

**Association of Reflexologists**
27 Old Gloucester Street
London
WC1N 3XX
Tel: 0990 673320

**The Breastfeeding Network**
P.O. Box 11126
Paisley
PA2 8YB
Tel: 0141 884 2472

**British Association for
Counselling**
1 Regent Place
Rugby
Warwickshire
CV21 2PJ
Tel: 01788 578328

**British Homoeopathic
Association**
27a Devonshire Street
London
W1N 1RJ
Tel: 0171 935 2163

**British Society of Medical and
Dental Hypnosis**
42 Links Road
Ashstead
Surrey
KT21 2HJ
Tel: 01372 273522

**Council for Acupuncture**
179 Gloucester Place
London
NW1 6DX
Tel: 0171 724 5756

**Council for Complementary and Alternative Medicine**
179 Gloucester Place
London
NW1 6DX
Tel: 0171 724 9103

**National Childbirth Trust**
Alexandra House
Oldham Terrace
Acton
London
W3 6NH
Tel: 0181 992 8637

**National Eczema Society**
163 Eversholt Street
London
NW1 1BU
Tel: 0171 388 5651
Fax: 0171 388 5882

**Register of Traditional Chinese Medicine**
19 Trinity Road
London
N2 8JJ
Tel: 0181 883 8431

## USA

**American Association of Naturopathic Physicians**
2800 East Madison Street
Suite 200
Seattle
Washington 98102
Tel: 206 323 7610

**American Holistic Medicine Association**
4101 Lake Boone Trail
Suite 201
Raleigh
North Carolina 27607
Tel: 919 787 5146

**Eczema Association for Science and Education**
1221 South West Yamhill
Suite 303
Portland
Oregon 97205
Tel: 503 228 4430

# Index